Loving the Soul Beneath the Autism

An Interior Analysis of the Impact a Special Needs Child Bestows upon the Family

Written By: Janele Hoerner

Edited By: Leslie Laird

Loving the Soul Beneath the Autism

Copyright © 2016 by Janele Hoerner

All rights reserved. No part of this book may be reproduced or transmitted in any form or by any means without written permission of the author.

Scripture quotations contained within this text are taken from The New American Bible Revised copyright © 1987 by World Bible Publishers, Inc.

This book is a means of expression from one single family's feelings on raising a child with special needs. It is not meant to be used as a means to diagnose another child exhibiting like symptoms, unless a doctor states that the like symptoms are factually accurate to obtain said diagnoses.

Formatting and cover design completed by the Author.

ISBN 10: 1516919017

ISBN 13: 978-1516919017

Written for all of the parents who feel alone and uncertain amongst the struggles of a newly diagnosed child. May you be led to a life of hope, acceptance, and a deeper love than you ever knew possible.

Acknowledgments

 First and foremost I would like to thank my loving and supportive husband who has never wavered from the person he was the first moment that I met him, which in itself is a rarity in the society in which we live. He is everything I had ever hoped to find in a husband, and I would not be the person I am today without him in my life. I would also like to thank each of my children who mold me every day into a more selfless individual as I constantly learn to think of another before myself. Although I began to change for the betterment of my first-born child's life, his impact is not any more exceptional than any of my other children's lives. I could write a complete book in the ways each of them has impacted not only my life but also the world in their own perfect and unique way.

 I would also like to thank my grandparents. They have had multiple titles in my life, and they swallowed what they wanted in their retirement years to raise a teenager who was less than what I should have been in many ways, but mostly in gratitude. Yet, I hope they understand how much they mean to me for everything they have done over the course of my own and my children's lives. I hope they understand all of the ways in which they have formed me as a person and how thankful I am for their constant in my lifetime. I would like to thank my Grandma Doris who was the first person to whom I expressed the desire to write a book. She encouraged me to do just that in order to help others.

 I would like to thank my mom who was emotionally there for me during my first-born's pregnancy when I felt entirely alone. She helped me begin my entrance back into bettering my life for the child who I was carrying as I returned to school shortly after my son was born. Although ending that career was misunderstood at the time, by not finishing my degree, my true calling was found in raising my children. I thank her for everything she attempted to do for my best interest. I am also thankful for my father, who has had many of his own battles in life and yet has risen above to become a recovering individual who understands that life is lived each moment at a time, one specific breath at a time. Thank you for working to better yourself to become the person I needed from a Daddy and now a Grandfather. You are both loved.

For my editor and high school teacher at Lancaster Catholic, Leslie Laird, who always promoted, guided, and believed in my writing from my first moments in her classroom. I would like to thank her for her happy personality, which also brought joy to an extremely difficult time in my life as well as currently going above and beyond her duty as a teacher to bring my dream into the book it has become. I am also grateful for another teacher of mine from the same high school. Mrs. Loretta Ferguson was a neighbor and eventually became a friend. She lived by example the life similar to the one I prayed that I would find. Thank you for your guidance, proof of concept that being a mother is the most important job there is to be done, and your will for my success.

To my son's first psychiatrist, Dr. Abonyi, who first diagnosed my son and brought us out of a life of confusion. I am thankful that she never ever grew tired of my endless questions as to why he had the conditions he did and all of her suggestions and understanding during the years of care. To Dr. Reis who currently works tirelessly to help us manage his medication and get the best services available for my son, and for the many children she works to help. Thank you for all you have done and continue to do to help families who feel alone with the children they have been gifted.

I am also thankful to the countless other individuals in my life who have formed me in both positive and negative ways, which unknowingly led me into the life I am currently proud to possess. Finally, this part would not be complete without stating that this book was not a work of my own, yet a work of God who planted an urgent feeling in me numerous Sundays, in no other place than the middle of church. May it be everything it is intended to be, and may I always be led to strive to become the individual who will one day be granted a home behind the heavenly gates.

Foreword

I'll never forget when my wife told me, "I'm writing a book about our son's autism." So many thoughts swirled through my head. Why would she want to do that? What makes her qualified for such a task? Mostly, however, I just wanted to know when she found the time. We have four children all under the age of seven, and, suffice it to say, they keep us very busy. I generally work long hours, so she really manages everything in our lives. I always refer to her as the Home Manager. She stays at home with the kids, pays the bills, takes care of all appointments, cooks, cleans, the laundry, everything. I, for one, know that the rare moment I get to myself would not be spent writing a book. As far as qualifications go, she's a fighter.

From the time we found out that our eldest son had high functioning autism, she's been a warrior for him. She's read countless books on the topic, constantly trying to improve her knowledge about the autism spectrum so she can help our son feel peace in the world. She knew he had some disadvantage in life when he was only two years old. I just thought he was a hyper mess. He was all over the place. I know a lot of parents feel that way, but this was different. Nothing held his attention for more than ten seconds…NOTHING. I rarely ever tried playing with him knowing it would end as soon as it started. It just wasn't fun. I always dreamed of teaching and playing tee-ball or baseball with my son when he was old enough to swing a bat. With Gracin, it was pointless. By the time I placed the ball on the tee, he was running away to do something else that would last but a moment. The more my wife read about autism, the more our lives changed.

She was always looking for a way to improve our son's life and inner peace. She was also trying to find better ways to just deal with him. He was a challenge on so many fronts. He argued about everything from the time he was twenty months old. I never met such a child who sometimes acted like a teenager.

So the idea of writing a book about our son, when we struggled so much with him, seemed a little hypocritical. We were by no means these saintly parents who were always patient and compassionate toward his every need. As I read her book, it dawned on me that that was not why she wrote it. We struggled, like I'm sure most parents with an autistic child do. We know all about the looks out in public when our son has a 45 minute meltdown from being overwhelmed. We understand that you just can't be calm at a restaurant because your child is a ticking time bomb. We would go to bed some nights feeling like the worst parents because of our lack of patience with him. We've always loved him dearly, but at times he was just difficult to deal with. He is so intelligent that we could never understand that he knew what $64 + 64$ was at the age of 3 but did not understand a simple request such as "please be quiet right now."

My wife wants other parents, grandparents, aunts, and uncles to understand that it's okay to admit the struggles, but love conquers the diagnosis. I'm not talking about a fluffy emotional kind of love but a true love that forfeits personal desires for the well being of the child. My wife and I have missed out on a lot of things that we would have loved to do so that our son would not feel inner turmoil. She writes this book not as a scientific doctor on autism, but as a loving mother who cherishes our son and would defend his rights to life, love, and happiness.

I could not be more proud of her. She is everything I wanted in a wife and mother for my children. She was determined to tell our story even if just one person found hope and help from what we have been through. She found the time to write this book, and not once did it affect our lives nor did she neglect me or the kids. I often tell her that she needs to take some time for herself, and the last three years that time was used for writing this book.

She offers this book so people may come to understand some of the struggles and joys of raising a child on the autism spectrum. We have found countless ways to help our son deal with the curveballs that life throws his way. Maybe other parents out there may find some ideas from her book to help their own children or someone they know who is on the spectrum. All children are unique, and those on the spectrum are no different. What works for one family may not work for another, but this book details some things we have found to help our son and ourselves. If you're a parent of a child who has autism and feel like you're failing as a parent, know that you're not alone. We have gone through many ups and downs raising our son, but at the end of each day, we try to reflect and acknowledge that we tried our best, and tomorrow we'll try again.

So enjoy, and peace be with you.

  Ryan Hoerner

Introduction: My Son's Disorder's Defined in my Own Words

Autism is a neurodevelopmental disorder that is categorized as a spectrum disorder. This means that all individuals given the diagnosis of autism fall within a range of high and low functioning individuals. The low functioning individual struggles with communicating through speech, as their language is limited. The high functioning individual often excels in the area of communication. This person has more social inabilities that result in being misunderstood by others because of looking typical in their appearance. For this book, I will only be speaking about high functioning individuals diagnosed with autism because that was the label given to my son, which was previously diagnosed as Asperger's.

Within the world of individuals struggling with high functioning autism as an everyday condition, there are a lot of misunderstandings. First and foremost is the misconception that these individuals are not empathetic. Although this can seem true to a spectator, it is not an inability to feel empathy that is part of the condition. This social disorder literally inhibits an understanding of how to communicate feelings and emotions. Although difficult to understand, a person with HFA does feel emotions and does want to help others who are feeling their own emotions. The problem is an inability to connect feelings to actions, requiring instruction in exactly how to act in each and every situation.

Socially, a person with HFA can come across as somewhat of a know it all. Because of their inability to understand social cues and without much instruction at an early age and beyond, that behavior may be the only way in which they understand how to step out of their shell and communicate with other individuals in the social world. As a developing child within the world, life is not in the least bit easy. For most children, at least knowing what to say to start a conversation is easy, knowing what to say when someone is crying is easy, and knowing when to believe someone is being nice or mean to is easy. To an autistic individual, nothing is concrete because while they think in black and white, the world thinks in a million different possibilities.

Life can be extremely overwhelming to these individuals because of all the sensory stimuli around them. A typical individual with high functioning autism does not understand that certain types of lights make buzzing noises, the computer makes a high pitched noise once it is turned on, the refrigerator makes a low hum, the furnace makes the floor vibrate, the wind can be intrusive as it blows and in different speeds without warning, birds chirp in different pitches, hugs can hurt as they provide either too much or too little stimuli by their variation, textures of clothing can feel as if they are attempting to scratch off the surface of one's skin, and the list goes on and on. Although it may seem as if these feelings are something every person in society deals with, to the individual with autism they are heightened to a level that causes sensory pain and so much discomfort that the person cannot function because of the level of distraction these sensitives produce.

Autism is often misunderstood and discounted as not being a real condition by some in the older generations. However, it is just as important as other special needs because the diagnosis provides a disability to the individual as a result of the neurodevelopmental condition. Although there is no cure for this condition, with the right early interventions by parents, extended families, and dedicated individuals in the form of doctors and therapists, the individual given the diagnosis can learn to understand why they are different, how to ease their sensitives, and how to embrace themselves as worthwhile individuals to the world around them.

Attention Deficit Hyperactivity Disorder (ADHD) is a neurobehavioral condition that affects more and more individuals each and every year just as autism does. It causes the affected individual to have the inability to sit still, relax, and focus on the task at hand for a substantial period of time. It causes harm to the individual themselves and the loved ones around them because their motor seems to never run out of gas, even in the middle of the night. It can produce problems with learning in school and behavior problems in all areas of one's life.

Although it is a separate condition from autism, itself, upwards of over half of all individuals with one diagnosis are given both diagnoses. The two conditions together can produce many fireworks for caretakers. With the right interventions and therapies, those with ADHD can be taught to fully function and learn to overcome the urge for constant movement.

Intermittent Explosive Disorder (IED) is also known as rage. Although this diagnosis is not commonly given to children, this was something that our family experienced all too well. Within what felt like a matter of seconds, our overly happy and smiling child would get a look of fear and defiance in his eyes mixed with anger. He would then unleash his inner monster on anyone within his space. It was out of the blue, shocking, and caused much pain to many of our family members yet was a critical part of his young life. Although now not given as a diagnosis to a child under six years of age according to the newest *DSM Manual of the American Psychiatric Association* (5th edition), it was a much-needed term for our son's young life. With time, patience, perseverance, constant monitoring, and medication, this too can be managed, and a person can rise above the diagnosis to recognize the feelings leading up to an occurrence as well as ways to divert misguided energy.

Please understand that I am not a doctor, and I do not have the background to explain in perfect detail any of these conditions other than my own experience. The descriptions above are simply my personal understandings of the specific diagnoses given to my son.

Preface

Loving the Soul Beneath the Autism can be read in two ways. You are encouraged to read the book in its entirety from front to back cover as you would a typical book. However, if you are a parent caring for your own special needs child, and you are exhausted with little time to spare, you can read only the first chapter of each individual part. Reading in this manner provides an overview as to what the author felt it was like parenting her child through each individual life stage. It also provides concise insight into how these parents transformed their lives as they were called by God to act in the precise way that their child needed. May you enjoy navigating through these pages as you are led into the exact life that you were meant to possess!

Table of Contents

Part 1: A Soul's Body in the Making
Chapter 1: Learning to Cherish Every Child 23
Chapter 2: Growing Contents 27
Chapter 3: He's Real 35
Chapter 4: Our Parenting Strategy was Love 39

Part 2: This Love it Seems is not Enough
Chapter 5: This Child Needs More Than I Can Give 46
Chapter 6: Rock My World Away 49
Chapter 7: A War on Sleep 55
Chapter 8: Rest, Peace, and the Correlation of Love........61

Part 3: The Overly Social Child
Chapter 9: The Blind Climb................................68
Chapter 10: A Mounting Paradox 73
Chapter 11: Becoming What I Always Envisioned 81
Chapter 12: Discovering Autism 85

Part 4: Not One, but Three Diagnoses
Chapter 13: A Violent Shaking...........................102
Chapter 14: Our Reset Button............................109
Chapter 15: Sensitivities, Frustration,
and Finally Enlightenment...............................119

Chapter 16: Not for the Weak of Heart 141

Part 5: Surrendering

Chapter 17: In Sight of the Summit.................................149
Chapter 18: Ready, Set, Let's Argue 155
Chapter 19: The Life I Discovered is Ever Changing 167
Chapter 20: Forever Imprinted 179

Part 6: The Supreme Gift of Perseverance

Chapter 21: The Magnificent Overlook 189
Chapter 22: Other's Blunt Opinions 195
Chapter 23: Becoming an Advocate...203
Chapter 24: Confessions Straight from a Mother's Heart........213

Appendix A: The Necessity of Sleep 224
Appendix B: Toilet Training 227
Appendix C: Family Explanation Letter 231
Appendix D: 1st Week of Medication......................................237
Appendix E: Sensory Integration Therapy 241

Part 1:
A Soul's Body in the Making

Chapter 1:
Learning to Cherish Every Child

Short of breath, I struggled to keep my head just above the salty water. Crashing waves pounded down over my shoulders while exhaustion began setting in over my entire body. I felt deserted. I mustered all the strength in my bones with one final act of desperation and sank down into the depths of the water. I found a huge rock sticking up from the ocean depths, and I pushed with all the energy in my being. In doing so, I was able to elevate my body through the brisk waters. As my head was guided to the top of a large wave, I let out a frantic scream into the atmosphere.

Scanning the coastline for help, I began to accept the inevitable path for my future. I watched as a dark triangle crept out of the water increasing its speed toward my exhausted body. Rain had begun to fall, and my heart was beating out of my chest. In my spiraling mental impairment, I felt the nudge of a large mass from under the dreary waters. Looking up towards the darkening sky, I began to pray from the depths of my soul as I felt myself being pulled down into the frigid waters.

I grasped my stomach in an ultimate attempt to save my unborn child even as I was repeatedly being dragged under the waves. I felt blood draining from my leg while I watched the shark let go of its hold and swim away. Leaving us to perish alone, but together, in the open water, I looked to God for both of our souls. Too tired to cry, scream, or even pray, we began to inevitably sink down into our demise.

Just as my body reached the ocean bottom, I felt a strong arm pull me above the water. A lifeguard had heard my smothered cries. Together we fought the strong storm that had blown in from deeper waters. I felt like the undertow had no intention of allowing us to reach the shore. We were caught in an almost inescapable cycle. The few individuals who were still on the beach waiting out the storm seemed clearly entertained by our endeavor. Their comments and gestures only distracted us from our mission.

Just as the waves finally started to calm, our repeated efforts pushed us onto the sandy beach. Collapsing into the shallow waves, we embraced each other in the newly warm sunlight. Although we did not yet have the strength to stand on our own two feet, we, thankfully, were on solid ground. The result of my almost cataclysmic end had bonded us together emotionally.

I looked around and wished I could happily lie on the dry and sandy beach, where I watched numerous parents laughing and playing with their babies. I loved the soothing sand in every aspect and desired to bask in the golden rays of the sun. I could not wait to watch my baby play at the water's edge while I enjoyed, in awe, his growth and development. I craved to play in the waves that hardly even reached my ankles, but that was not the course our lives had taken. Over time, I found meaning in my almost destructive experience, because it was in those darkest hours that I learned all about life's true meaning.

♥

Autism, High Functioning to be exact, combined with ADHD and Intermittent Explosive Disorder were our large ocean waves and violent storm. Combined together, their severity could have been our destruction, but we would not have them capsize our lives. Moment by moment, we, as parents, pushed on until the waves were no longer knocking us from our feet. With what seemed like the world against us, my future husband and I battled through an almost impossible forecast.

Even though I had made some immature decisions to land my child and myself in a deep ocean, a wonderful man pulled us to safety. That man came to our rescue in one of my darkest moments, seven months into my pregnancy. Within time, my shark, which had helped create this child, swam away. He had hurt my hope and spirit with his bite, yet he allowed us the time to heal as I married the lifeguard who pulled my child and me to safety. Together my husband and I confronted our son's impending behaviors while holding on tight to our little boy, who we loved so dearly.

It was by the love of our son's soul, which lay buried beneath his neurological diagnosis, that we learned how to truly cherish each and every child. May you find hope in our true story, encouragement in our techniques, and a deep love for the soul of all special needs children. For it is by the love of the least, the bruised, and the smallest of all humans that we find the greatest love in this selfish world. Slowly but surely, my perfect, wanted, and wonderful child became my fighting reason for everything in life. Yet, I want you to come to know the entire story. So, before I begin to elaborate further, let me start at the beginning, to the day when I first realized I was carrying a little child inside of me.

Chapter 2:
Growing Contents

E veryone knows that saying, "Be careful what you wish for." Well my wish came true on a typical Thursday morning...

That morning began like every other weekday morning that preceded it, with my phone alarm clock singing at 6 a.m. As I hit the off button, I rolled over and closed my eyes once again. 6:15 came far too quickly as the second wake-up song began. After hitting the silencing button once again, I laid back on the bed staring at my fan. In my half asleep daze-like-state, I began to dream a few years into the future. I dreamt of a loving husband and little children playing together, laughing, and jumping into their parents' bed. Just as I began turning my head to see the face of my adoring husband, the final commencing of the 6:30 buzzing began radiating throughout the room.

By now, I was late, as usual. I placed my feet into my fuzzy purple flip-flop slippers and grabbed a towel as I headed for the shower. Just as I left the room, I turned back remembering the box that was hidden under my mattress for safekeeping. I slowly pulled out the special package and folding it secretly into my towel I hurried off to get ready for my day. I headed down the freezing steps quietly and peered out the kitchen window where it was a cold 17 degrees.

Arriving at my girly, perfumed bathroom affixed with every purple accessory that I could find, I turned up the heat. When I opened the annoying squeaky door, I was immediately hit with a soothing aroma of lavender. It always had the ability to put me in an uplifting mood. I excitedly pulled the hidden box from my towel and carefully took out the contents, with anticipation, of the possibly perfect future ahead of me. I carefully laid my used pregnancy test on the bottom right corner of the sink as I swiftly showered.

I had the intention of not peeking at the results until my shower was over, but my determined and overly obsessed mind conquered my will. Soon enough I was pulling back the curtain to read that one tiny word that I always imagined seeing. That one word brought so much joy to my thoughts. It was honestly the only thing that I ever passionately thought about in my twenty years. Finally, I saw them, the eight letters that I was convinced would change my life forever: PREGNANT!

I must have pulled that shower curtain back five or six more times just to make sure that I did not miss another small, but just as important, word NOT. Except there continued to only be one word in my view. Feeling as if I was floating in midair, with not one ounce of fear in my mind, I was elated that my growing contents were not a figment of my imagination. I was, in fact, carrying a tiny and very special little child. In that moment, I was entirely consumed with the thoughts of this precious baby growing in my womb. I literally could not stop smiling! I was in love and so filled with excitement that I had not the faintest idea that I would never again be the same person who got out of bed that morning.

Thinking back to my own childhood just a bit, I reminisced how all I ever wanted was my own baby or a sister. I had baby dolls upon baby dolls, and every girl name that I could think of, my baby was named. Each time she was dropped, I got to name her again and start over. It was the magical obsession of my childhood mind. I knew, no I was convinced, that I was destined to have little girls of my own and a lot of them. I never even considered that I could have a little boy.

As I aged, when people asked how many children I wanted, my answer was always six. Since I was an only child and my grandmother had six, I felt I needed that pattern to continue. Patterns were always very important to me, so six sounded like the perfect but non-negotiable number. From a very early age, I knew that I wanted children. I only needed to find the guy who shared my same passion. I just never knew finding the ideal husband would be so incredibly hard.

Unfortunately, I would soon learn that I was going to be alone in my happiness about this child. Caught in the moment with a hopeful excitement of the unknown, I paused for a moment to send a text to the father of my unborn child. I simply wrote that I would be over after I got off work that night and closed my phone. I know I never received a response back from him, but I did not think anything of it at the time.

Driving to work that morning, I noticed how cautious I was. Skipping my morning iced coffee stop brought an even bigger smile to my face as I fought the traffic rush. Arriving at work that morning, I was in such a happy state-of-mind, that I could not even contain myself. As I opened the door and greeted the child for whom I was a nanny, his mother must have known something was different. She jokingly asked where my Frappuccino was. Smiling from ear to ear, I replied that I did not have time to stop! Knowing me better than I apparently knew my own patterns, she pushed further.

Ignoring her prying remarks, I picked up her little baby and envisioned how close I was to picking up my own child. My mind was running circles around itself, and it was in that moment that everything came crashing down. This was so much bigger than I could ever have imagined. I needed help. Sadly, but somewhat ironically, before this all I cared about was having a baby. I had not even considered the facts of supporting that new life. I froze with her son in my hands, and I wept. I could not stop my mouth from rambling every thought in my skull. The whole story came spewing out. The tears poured down my cheeks as I confessed to her that I felt completely alone! The reality of my life was that I had no real way to take care of a tiny baby on my own.

I lived with my Grandparents and was working my way through nursing school at the time. I had no extra money to my name, no money for a house, clothes, toys, or anything for this child. I was so incredibly blinded by just wanting what I wanted, that I allowed myself to have a child with someone I was engaged but not married to. He had used what I desired so badly to get what he wanted from me. I knew he did not want a family like I wanted, and in acknowledging that, I only cried harder.

At last she interrupted my tears to speak. Her words made me cringe. I began to feel sick while listening to all of her opinions, which honestly made total sense, until she said the final word that hurt to my core. That one strong word that I did not want to hear: abortion. I knew that someone would mention it. I just never thought it would come from the mouth of a mother I admired. In that instance, all of the respect I had for her left. Her theory, as she explained, was that I should enjoy my twenties and then have children after I discovered who I truly was.

I always knew, though, that I wanted to be a mom. I loved being a nanny and knew I would love, even more, being a mother. So in hearing those words roll off her tongue, I was offended with every ounce of my being. In an overly emotional state, I knew I had to leave my job and get away from anyone who would even talk about that word. In my opinion, I had already made my decision by allowing this baby to come into existence, and now it was this child's life. A life, I felt, I was not privileged to end, even if that meant my own life would have to drastically change.

After quitting my job, I was scared to death to tell anyone. I drove straight to the local doctor who accepted pregnant women without insurance. Later, following what seemed like an eternity and a pile of paperwork, I was seen for an initial appointment. My options were presented to me, and I set up my 1st ultrasound.

The obvious next step, it seemed, was to go and see the guy who shared this wonderful idea of having a baby before marriage. Although I was so excited to tell him what I thought was good news, I just knew in the pit of my stomach that he could reject me and this child too. I was scared. Pulling into the driveway, I was shaking. I think I sat in the car for ten minutes just playing with the ring that I imagined was going to be taken off of my finger in a matter of a few words. Even though the word abortion was never used, I quickly realized that I was all alone.

A week later, I went to my 1st ultrasound with my only support person at my side: my mom. I was experiencing a total rush of emotions while I saw and heard my child's heartbeat. I was elated with joy, envisioning my glorious little baby. Yet, my future seemed so bleak at the same time. My pregnancy was officially confirmed, and my due date was set for November 15th, 2008. I was ecstatic to have this child who I had always craved, but craving was all it was. I now sat witnessing a remarkable moment in my life with my mom at my side instead of a loving and supportive husband. The image of the life that I thought I would have was turned upside down as reality hit me.

The first trimester of my pregnancy proved to be harder than my wildest dreams. I was exhausted and miserable. I had constant headaches, and I got dizzy every time I stood up. Needless to say, nothing stayed in my stomach for long. Morning sickness became an understatement because I was sick all day and all night. I only found relief in Turkey Hill Coke Slushies, but only if I was sucking it constantly through the straw. I knew that the soda was not good for the baby. I tried to limit them to one a day, but eventually my Grandmother, who was a nurse, put a stop to my daily habit. I traded it for ginger pieces, which just made me gag more. I counted the hours until the second trimester started when I was told my sickness would end. The morning sickness ending was only wishful thinking as twelve weeks came and went.

To my disbelief, at the start of my 13th week, I felt a surprising sensation in my stomach, which turned out to be my baby's first kick. Although it was very early, my midwife told me that anything was possible. I might be feeling the flutters of the child because I was so sensitive. It was amazing! I could push on my stomach at any point, and, within seconds, I would feel the flutters in that exact place. That flutter gradually became a kick that I begged to be calmed. I was kicked, drummed, stretched, and hurt from inside with no relief. My baby was a boy, and he kicked with a vengeance. These movements were so hard that they would make me throw up, and I had no relief from morning sickness throughout my second trimester. The kicks brought on pre-term contractions that landed me in the hospital several times. I spent multiple nights in the triage of the hospital having medicine pumped into my IV.

As the second trimester came to a close, I was in an unbreakable pattern of sleeping, studying, and visiting the hospital.

I held on to the thought of a family for this baby as hard as I could during those first two trimesters until the engagement ring was removed from my finger. Leaving me standing alone in my driveway, I watched as my little boy's father drove away. I watched and I watched and I pleaded with God, but his car never turned around. He had made up his mind, and my futile attempts at changing it were of no use. Feeling week and dizzy, I sat on the hard driveway until it was dark. I was inconsolable over the next few weeks as I realized the full weight of being alone. I had actually believed the lies that a boy will tell a girl to get what they want. I vowed to never allow another person to hurt me the way that he had. I had given that boy everything of meaning to me, when in reality he deserved nothing to begin with. What was I to do now?

The start of my third trimester seemed to be manageable. I was learning to function pretty well until the one night that changed everything. I must have let out a scream in my sleep that was enough to wake up my Grandmother. I was soon back in the hospital, and the next thing I knew, I was admitted into labor and delivery. At 31 weeks I was having steroid shots injected into my legs to develop my child's lungs because my contractions would not stop with any of the hospital's measures. Finally, after three days, with no relief from steady seven to ten minute contractions, a new medicine relieved the pain. The medicine relaxed my uterus, and the contractions were thankfully gone. I was released from the hospital and put on bed rest for the remainder of my pregnancy.

Chapter 3:
He's Real

My pregnancy, up until my seventh month, was nothing close to happy. Although unknown to me, the future was just about to open up. By the grace of God, I was introduced to a very sweet and caring man who understood how deeply I needed a friend. Even though he was only a friend, our daily talks gave me something to focus on, other than my sickness. With the sight of my son in mind, I developed a true friendship with no hidden agendas for the first time in my life. As time progressed, without the intention of it, we both felt drawn to each other as we discovered similarities. I kept my walls up out of fear, but for some reason he kept wanting to spend time with me.

Even though I felt nauseous until the day of my delivery, it did not seem as bad now that I felt worth something instead of feeling like a piece of trash to be discarded. I had my 13th ultrasound at my 38th week checkup and was told that I had a healthy child getting ready for his debut. I was able to stop my medication, and I felt great for the first time in my pregnancy. I was now able to leave the house again. I felt free!

The constant rolling and kicking inside me brought great joy during the next few weeks as I anticipated my first-born son's arrival. I went on my first official outing with my newfound friend, and he poured out his heart and soul to me. I was in total shock that anyone could be interested in a girl in my current state. I was ready to deliver a baby any day, one that he had no obligations to care for, yet he wanted both of us, and that baffled me. As he kissed my baby bump and told my little boy that he would take care of him no matter what, I felt a rush of feelings. In my own fear, torn as to what I should do or say, I pulled away. In my mind, I questioned everything. How could I begin a relationship with someone right now? How would I feel if it did not work out? The questions continued to gnaw at my mind. I did not want my son to experience any more pain than I had already bestowed upon him.

The first snow of the year marked the day of my anticipation. I arrived at Labor and Delivery as my contractions were getting progressively closer together. I was moved into my own birthing room. This was it! The moment was here. I was in pain but ecstatic. I knew within the next few hours I would be holding my little child, a boy, whose name was yet to be determined.

The moments that followed were nothing short of remarkable. In one instance, feelings of love, excitement, compassion, and a healthy fear were flooded into my exhausted mind. It was unfathomable to me that this tiny 6 lb. 12 oz. child grew inside my body for the last 41 weeks. Witnessing him take his first few breaths was spectacular. His skin was so wrinkly, warm, and soft! His head was perfectly round with tiny remnants of blonde hair. His eyes were a deep emerald green. I felt complete with him in my arms.

This child was mine, and I was solely responsible for his upbringing. There I was, 21 years old, holding this tiny baby, with no real idea of who I even was as a person. I was so young, so incredibly unaware of all of the situations that were going to unfold in the next few years. In that moment, though, I felt peace

He's Real

and love. The one and only thing I knew I could offer this child was my dedication to become the best mother that I could be, and that is exactly what I was determined to do.

Gracin was welcomed into this world on November 22nd at 6:23 a.m. He was my saving grace, so the name fit perfectly, and my first day with him was pure bliss. He was so content to lie in my arms. He barely opened his eyes to look around before drifting back into a dreamland. He mostly just slept cuddled in my arms. He was perfect!

His first night the nurse came in to check on us almost every hour because I was a new mom. Each time she patiently asked me to place him back into that plastic bin that they called a cradle. I tried my best to listen to her advice, but as soon as she left the room, I promptly picked him back up into the secure fit of my arms. I felt as though he was the puzzle piece that I was always missing. After years of yearning for these moments, I was not going to miss any part of the experience. I could not understand how she thought I would be so negligent to drop him as I slept. I could not sleep. I did not want to miss any moment of his existence.

Night became morning, and Gracin celebrated his first day in the world. Time sped by. We were discharged from the hospital. We celebrated Thanksgiving five days after he was born. The entire holiday had more meaning than ever before. Two days later, he had a week-old portrait taken. My precious sleeping child was draped on my chest as I kissed the top of his tiny head. That moment will never leave my mind. Standing there in awe, viewing his adorable sleeping face in digital format, I held back the tears. How was this child already a week old? I was overwhelmed by all of the firsts he was already making. His first yawn, first day, first hiccup, and first week already gone by. Time really does fly once you focus on an individual other than yourself.

As time passed, I noticed he rarely cried. I believed it was because I was attentive to his every need. He slept almost constantly and was held day and night. The first time he let out a real cry was during his first bath. At the time, I believe I cried almost as much as he did, realizing that I could not save him from everything, even though it was only water. I was completely dedicated to this little child, but this was the first of many times that I would come to realize that I could not help him through all of life's problems. I saved that little umbilical cord tip as a reminder that at one time he was attached to me and lived because of me though now it would be because of my teaching example that he would grow and learn in the world to be the child, teenager, and adult that he was made to be.

Chapter 4:
Our Parenting Strategy was Love

With each day that passed, I was beginning to realize the actual depth of the decision I had chosen for not only me but also for this small child. The tan mark from my engagement ring was almost gone as Christmas approached and Gracin's "father" was proving to fall into a slowly dissipating pattern. My heartstrings ached for my infant son. Initially, when Gracin was born, he came to see him three times a week for a few hours. However, by the third month, he showed his face barely once a week. He had a new girlfriend, and this baby was clearly not the most important person in his life. As time pushed on, he faded more and more and eventually stopped seeing us altogether for reasons I may never fully understand.

I, on the other hand, had been given one of the best gifts I could have ever imagined. I was certainly not going to let this guy beat me down any longer though I still was leery of trusting anyone again. Yet, a new man had been placed in my life before Gracin's birth, and the harder I tried to just be friends with him, the more I saw he was so much more than a friend. He had literally stepped up to become a daddy overnight and took on that task with open arms. He was everything that I had always wanted but never felt I would find. He was always with us when he was not working.

He was the best friend that I never had. His promises proved true, and I began to see that he was what I needed in all aspects.

I fought an internal battle acknowledging that I could not be a parent alone, wanting to trust again, but being scared because I was choosing for both my son and myself. I did not want my future children to have different fathers. I didn't want a broken family. Trying to let go of my faults and not focus on the past, I resolved to make sure the next time I trusted, it would be forever. I wanted not only a father for my son but also a real daddy who adored and wanted the best for my child. I wondered if this guy was going to get sick of us too. Letting go of my fears, I trusted in him. When Gracin was 6 months old, this incredible man knelt down to ask me the question that solidified all of the thoughts of my mind.

I deeply believed that although my future husband had no ties to Gracin's blood, he thought of him as a son. That was exactly what we needed in order to start our lives as a true family. Two months later Gracin said "Dada" for the first time. At that point, there was no reluctance in my mind. From the heart of a little child who had heard his voice from inside the womb on a consistent basis, with no prompting on my part, who was I to argue with what name Gracin provided him? I knew in my heart that my husband-to-be was sent by God in my darkest moments to save not only my life but my little son's life as well. The point to all of this is that we never referred to him as my son or your son; he was our son, and we raised him together. Not many people even knew that Gracin was not from this man's bloodline because to us, it did not need to be announced. This was our child, and that was how we were going to live.

Our parenting strategy did have to change over time as we realized that our son was not developing typically. It never occurred to us at first because there was no diagnosis presented at birth for his condition. It was an evolving revelation over time that we had to accept and help our families accept also. The existence of this child was enough to fight for, and fight is what we did.

As any parent knows, the first few weeks of raising a child can be downright tiring. Time blends together, and sleep eludes the best of parents. Everyone reassured me that with time my little boy would sleep longer and deeper, but it just never happened. At six weeks of age, he was only sleeping for a twenty-minute nap three times a day. My wonderful and devoted Daddy-in-the-making walked him back and forth for at least an hour every night so Gracin could fall asleep. After he left for the night, Gracin would wake up every single hour, on the hour, to eat. I felt as though as soon as I was done feeding, I was waking up to feed again.

Nights were miserable to say the least. Gracin was having trouble digesting breast milk, which was supposed to be the most easily digested substance for a baby. We were constantly rubbing his tiny tummy, moving his little legs, and feeding him gas drops to ease his discomfort. He hated being put down and would cry, sucking in more air leading to almost constant hiccups, which led to more air being trapped in his belly. I felt he was just colicky, and, being a new mom, I really did not think anything of his seemingly extra needs. I knew he was not an easy baby, but since he was content with being held, nothing more crossed my mind.

As life continued, one thing resonated in my mind and deeply troubled me. Gracin was almost four months old, and he never smiled. He always seemed to have a curious look to his facial features but never a smile. I used to refer to him as my little grumpy old man, but I craved to see that smile. Gracin would, in fact, smile in his sleep (so I knew he was capable), but why not while he was awake?

That glorious moment finally arrived at 4 months and 3 weeks of age. I was ecstatic. Well, as life goes, with one problem out of the way, another one was on the horizon, and this one was not as easy as a smile. Feeling overwhelmed by his twenty-minute cat naps, now only twice a day, and feeding every hour throughout the night, I did not know what to do. I wanted to be able to place him in his bed for at least an hour to sleep, and I did not feel that was unreasonable given his age.

Each day he slept less and less. I could not place him down in a bed, swing, or anything without waking him. Many people told me being held so much was spoiling him, but I tried not to pay attention to the advice of others. He continued to be a very light sleeper, and no one could be quiet enough during his brief naps. We bought various noise machines and mobiles, but the slightest change in the music would wake him. I tried everything to extend his sleep. Nothing worked. I even broke down and bought my first parenting book to help babies sleep without tears. After trying everything in this five-star reviewed book with little to no success, I gave up for a time on parenting books. I was too tired to read anyway.

I wanted to spend any free time I had with my son now that I was back in school, so I relied on my own senses to figure out what I felt was right for my child. I managed pretty well to retain my perfect grade point average, even in my sleep-deprived state. In my mind, being a nurse was the only way to support us. I had no intention of fully relying on anyone to take care of us again.

I tried my best to relax and play with my little child, but his attention span was fleeting. He had no interest in toys that did not make noise as they only seemed to bore him. He was in love with things he could turn on and off or watch spin; although, even those would not keep his interest for long. While he was switching things on and off, he seemed happy, even though after a while, his eyes would get very big and glazed over. It was as if he was over stimulating himself by all of the noise and movement. He then would scream an ear-piercing scream until my eardrums felt as if they were going to burst. I did not know what was going on with my little child. The pictures of Gracin at those stages actually show a very confused little boy. At the time, I just thought he wanted more attention. It was almost as if he was begging for someone to calm him down.

Eventually I seemed to get immune to the loss of sleep, and life proceeded. Gracin hit every milestone on time, if not early, and often surprised us with his knowledge. He was such a very busy child. Not a toy in the world would hold his attention for more than thirty seconds. As early as nine months, we were convinced he knew his basic colors because every time we asked him to crawl to a specific colored block, he would. He held it above his head with a smile as if to say, "Look what I did." Hundreds of times, throughout his ninth month, he repeated this and was never wrong, not even one time. We did not think much of it, other than it being a cute attribute. He was already saying "Dada" and "Mama" at this time. Surprisingly, at only ten months the words evolved into two and three word sentences like, "Mom ball get," "Dada up now," and "I love you." The words were stated clear as clear could be and just rambled out of his mouth. He loved talking and had no intention of stopping. Impressed with his abilities at less than a year of age, we made sure to write down his achievements so not to forget, but really we were just thankful the ear-piercing screaming had stopped.

The facts as they were, I was already exhausted by the time his eyes opened in the morning. Being so busy in my own life with school, planning a wedding, and buying our first house, I just pushed forward. Our ultimate goal was not for raising the smartest kid on the block, it was simply for raising this child to one day enter into a heavenly paradise. Even though we desired to have a well behaved child, as anyone else does, we did not want to break his will by forcing him to fit into a set of rigid standards for his development.

I did in fact become, for the first time in my life, very envious of others. Mothers with babies around Gracin's age would talk with such love and admiration as their children sat by their feet playing with the same pair of keys for what felt like an eternity. I, on the other hand, could not even fully sit on a chair before chasing after my little one, who laughed at any instruction I gave him. I would hear of babies sleeping through the night as I attempted to smile hoping to God they did not ask what my nights were like. I was embarrassed, exhausted, and overwhelmed as to what I was doing wrong. I kept telling myself that all I needed to do was love my son for who he was, and it would all come together as he aged. Although, as he got older, it became so much harder to simply love.

Part 2:

This Love it Seems is not Enough

Chapter 5:
This Child Needs More Than I Can Give

Lying motionless on the edge of the ocean, with no breath left in my lungs, I felt the tide begin to recede. My body felt like a weighted anchor in the saturated sand as I attempted to crawl from the path of the waves. Falling into the dry sand, I again collapsed onto my back while the healing rays of the sun began to warm my drained being.

Moving ever so slightly, I repositioned the tiny new child in my arms feeling him hug me in his sleep. The gentle wind gusts felt soothing given the humid temperatures as I gazed down smiling at the tiny hairs moving upon his bald head. All felt perfect. I sensed a light mist fall down from the darkening clouds above. With not a care in the world, I closed my eyes, curling up closer to the warm body beside me who had just saved our lives. Embracing the feelings of love, relaxation, and warmth, I allowed my body to rest for the time being.

Opening my eyes once again to look out over the glistening waters, I watched in awe as the plum and sapphire clouds began to put the sun to sleep over the restless ocean. Movement diverted my attention from the waves as my child awoke. With a smile and a giggle, he tottered away on his own two feet. His little footprints

This Child Needs More Than I Can Give

led straight to the water's edge. Together we watched him run, play, and jump within the ocean waves. Bringing my body into an upright position, I gazed into the upper atmosphere thanking God for this newfound second chance.

Approaching my laughing little prince, I braced myself as he darted off in the opposite direction. Laughing excitedly, he found enjoyment in this unending game of tag. Calling his name into the wind, I began to lose enjoyment, as I briefly paused to playfully pat the sand. Encouraging him to come back to me, yet acknowledging his own free will, I let out a sigh and began to chase him down the coast. Running off in the direction of the sunset, I followed a path of toes pressed into the sand. Scrambling all the faster, I watched as his little body gained more distance from me than I was comfortable with. Dashing at full pace, I exuded the rest of my energy in seeing him approach a pier of rocks.

He climbed onto the rocks to escape my grasp. Just as I reached him, his leg slipped into a crevice. Freeing him into the safety of my arms, he pushed away as I spun him around and around. Falling dizzily onto the sand, we laughed while he proceeded to tackle me into the rushing waves. Standing up to escape an incoming swell, I watched as his tiny feet continued to spin about. Feeling as though I had won my fight and caught my lifeline, I picked up my little one in all of his perfection and continued to spin and spin.

♥

With no direct recognizable signs of a special need for the majority of our son's first two years, we were initially at a loss for what was going on with our growing child. We sensed that something was different, yet we did not have the faintest idea how to help him. I wanted to believe that all my child needed was a good night's sleep, but that did not change his behavior patterns as I had hoped.

We attempted to implement every typical behavior modification strategy that we could think of, but nothing worked as was suggested. He made us look ridiculous in public, as we ran after this child who endlessly laughed at any instruction we gave him. He drew everyone's glances, acting as the center of attention while we tried to control a seemingly typical child. At a loss of what we should do, with a child who exhausted any adult more than one child ever should, we felt out of options. We held out hope that as his age increased, he would calm down. So, as life pressed forward, we continued to chase, laugh, and spin with Gracin. Desperately we attempted to enjoy his constant movement, but day in and day out, his game was no longer entertaining.

With an intense examination of his behaviors and more devotion to him as a person, we may have caught on sooner, but in being so young ourselves and caught up in our own lives, we missed the signs. I always believed that love, expressed through words and hugs and combined with gentle guidance, were all that was needed to raise a well-rounded child, but we were not raising a typical child. Our child was developing differently to no fault of our own, even though all eyes were on us to control our rambunctious toddler. We strived each day to surround him with love as countless as the grains of sand at the ocean. Inevitably we had to accept that our love was not enough. As time proceeded, we discovered that not only were we on a journey to discover the neurological conditions developing in his brain but also what the word love truly meant after all.

Chapter 6:
Rock My World Away

Love was all I wanted to give. I desired to cradle my little child and read endless stories on our couch, play at the park for hours, and take quiet walks while we discovered the world together. Nothing about our lives was quiet and peace-filled though. Those quiet walks I craved were exhausting because our son refused to sit in a stroller, let alone to take a breath between words. The toys that mounted around him and equipment at the park bored him, as he would rather collect sticks, then count, and throw them. Those books I wanted to read my child were whipped from my grasp after the first page, in the time that he was scrambling off to the next thing. I shed multiple tears over the life I believed I had wanted but was drained by.

At the time of his 1st birthday, I was so proud of what we had endured thus far and where we were headed in our lives. We rented out a venue to celebrate this wonderful child's year on earth, and all of our close family attended. With my mom's help, I made multiple cakes, each in the shape of a letter in his name. Gracin sat in the center of the room, at the head of a table, happily digging into the first piece of cake. He had an intense look of happiness mixed with over-stimulation in his eyes, as he viewed it as his mission to make everyone laugh hysterically at him.

He truly captivated the utmost attention of everyone at the party, responding to any requests that were made of him. I had never seen a baby hold a crowd's attention as he did that day. He talked on and on to everyone with his extensive vocabulary using some of his favorite terms like screwbiby (screwdriver), whateber (whatever), and DaddynMama (his one word combination created for us). He always made you feel special being in his presence. It was an amazing day and marked the beginning of his next stage of development.

After the effect of the year one celebration concluded, life went back to a somewhat normal, yet chaotic, state. Our lives were busy as I was taking care of Gracin, attending classes, planning a wedding, and helping to renovate our future home. With my child in tow for almost all of my endeavors, there was very little down time. The time I did schedule into our day for rest, was really just me fighting with him to lie down and sleep.

As the effects of not sleeping were starting to take their toll on my body, I watched as my appetite left, my body dropped to an unhealthy weight, and I got dizzy upon any physical exertion. Throughout the night, during the one-hour increments of sleeping, I laid propped up on my bed with a pillow continuously nursing my child. With one arm I held his body as he fed in his sleep, and with the other I studied with a tiny light illuminating my book or computer.

I believed in breastfeeding on demand, but after following what I thought was best for him, I began to realize it had to be best for me also. I could not break his latch without waking him up, and he would not fall asleep without nursing in my arms. I was left baffled at how this arrangement was somehow working for my tiny son because I felt like I was living in a fog.

Rock My World Away

One sleepless night I gave in to a late night impulse buy when an ad popped up on my computer screen. It was an oversized rocking chair with room for two. It had plush seating and a matching rocking ottoman, which in my mind could double as a bed. To my dismay, this chair did not lead to Gracin sleeping more; however, upon his hourly awakening, all I had to do was start rocking to help him drift back to sleep without his eyes opening. As a result, I received just a little more sleep, and I also discovered how much this little boy cherished being rocked.

Therefore, rocking became a huge part of our daily routine, and I was filled with some well-deserved quiet moments where I could simply hold and cherish my busy little boy. Reclining in our chair, he would lie still as could be for a minute or two as I gently swayed back and forth. This bonding time was heaven sent in my time of need to experience calm with my child, even if it was only for such short periods of time.

Although, as life happened and time passed, the rocking-chair-quiet was not enough to hold his interest. It began to bore him, and I needed to find something to extend those sessions of sitting peacefully with Gracin throughout the day. At first I tried watching TV with him or reading books, but those activities did not hold his interest in the least bit. I tried playing games like Patti Cake and singing nursery songs, but they just stimulated him all the more.

In one final attempt to extend these elements, I began to pray out loud while I tussled his hair with my fingers. At first, he pushed my hand away and started to get down, but he quickly turned his body around and said, "Sing again." With tears in my eyes, I placed Gracin beside me once again and began to sing some prayers to him.

In observing my Grandmother say her prayers later that day, I watched again as my little child climbed into her lap to rock with her. I observed how the meditations combined with the continuous rocking motion calmed his restless being. Her prayers did not change in tone. As a result, they were the perfect things for Gracin. In picking up a Rosary that night, I sat with my son as I started singing the same recitation of prayers as my Grandmother had. Immediately, Gracin repeated the prayers with me, and as I gazed down at his tiny fingers grasping the beads, I was in awe at the moment I was just given.

After that God-given experience, I sat down in the rocking chair with him three times a day with the hope that we could get through the entire Rosary - about 15 minutes - without him jumping down. I felt so blessed to have such a wonderful little boy who seemed to be more devoted to prayer than I had recently been. In those quiet moments, as I would watch his chest slowly rise and fall and feel his fast-beating heart against my body, I would attempt to sing as slowly as possible. I wanted those moments to last just a few seconds longer before he was sliding down off of my lap. Each day as he slid down off of the chair and rounded the corner to the next thing, before I could even get to my feet, numerous questions flooded my mind. I would question why my son would sit still only for this particular time? Why could we not also sit and read an entire children's book while rocking? Why did he move so fast and dart around like a racket ball thrown against the wall? Did I do something to make him like this?

I had been around at least a couple dozen children around his age in my life, and not one of them behaved as he did. All of those babies and young toddlers fell asleep in their mother's arms with little to no effort. They could then be placed either in their crib, a swing, or a bed, and there they would remain asleep for another hour or even two. Why was this child not the same? I could count on one hand how many times Gracin had been asleep in his crib.

He could never be put down after falling asleep in your arms; he required you to also take a nap with him attached to you. This child was complex. He was unique. Gracin, in my opinion, was just plain exhausting. As the thoughts continued to envelop my mind, one thing was for sure, repetition was the key for calming this child, and I was thankful to find that the Rosary was the perfect answer for us.

Chapter 7:
A War on Sleep

As my frustration grew and mounted with Gracin's lack of sleep, I began to feel hopeless. I had so many opinions coming at me from many different sources, and I was downright confused. I never would have thought that a child's sleep patterns needed to be examined in as much depth as I was doing now. I wanted to believe that my child did not have to cry in order to sleep for a continuous period, but no matter what I tried, his sleep was not extending beyond 45 minutes in duration. After much research, anticipation, and tears shed on the topic, I purchased a new book with a happy little sleeping baby on the front. It is called *Healthy Sleep Habits, Happy Child*, written by Dr. Marc Weissbluth, who presents three different ways to help a child sleep (See Appendix A: The Necessity of Sleep).

This is the only book that I found showing multiple strategies in helping a child sleep. It also explains why sleep is such an important factor in raising a child. I read this book from front to back multiple times before implementing any of the techniques suggested.

The 13th chapter examines unrestricted breastfeeding. Weissbluth states that, "To maintain or develop healthy sleep habits for your child, have the courage to do what is best for the child." For some reason this sentence resonated in my foggy viewpoint as I began to believe that I had to become courageous, something I always lacked, in order to help my child sleep. Although I wanted Gracin to sleep through the night, I did not want to break the mother and baby bond that I believed in. I wanted him to feel that I would do whatever he needed for his comfort, but living without sleep, in the patterns our lives had fallen into, had to end. He was not outgrowing this life stage of development.

After careful consideration of my son's health and a full month of weighing our options, I picked the method I felt was best for us. At that point in our lives, I felt I needed to help him sleep soundly, and I was convinced some initial tears could not break the bond between us. In following the advice of a doctor deeply committed to helping children sleep well for proper brain development and who believed in having a well-rested family above all, we embarked on our new start. In addition, since I was already learning about the anatomy of the body in nursing school, I knew that the physiology of the brain was at the root of the proper functioning for the rest of the body. I felt like I had wasted too many months allowing my child to not sleep deeply, and, as I was his mother, it was my job to help him function the best he could.

Following what was suggested did not mean I had to stop breastfeeding my child on demand during his waking hours or even to an almost sleep-like state at night. It just meant that he did not have to rely on my breast for his only comforting technique. He could use his own body to feel security also. I wanted my child to depend on me and know I was the utmost devoted to him, but I did not have to continue to give him all of my energy anymore.

Since the two of us were not functioning where we should be, I believed that in choosing the quickest method outlined in Dr.

A War on Sleep

Weissbluth's book, we could be sleeping better and faster. I questioned my motives many times to make sure I was not doing this selfishly, out of my own pure desperation for sleep. I did not believe I would ever become the mother who let her child cry for no reason, but reading the pages over and over helped me remember why I was doing this practice.

I reminded myself that all babies cry, and sometimes they even cry when nothing is wrong. Gracin, on the other hand, never cried, so a few tears could not hurt. Before the start of the first night on his new journey of self-soothing, I rocked with him and prayed an entire Rosary with him by my side. I asked God to help us through this tough process while he entered into an almost drowsy state. As I carried him to his crib, I told him I loved him and gave him his tiny puppy blanket before saying goodnight.

Before I even had time to shut the door, he was already standing up attempting to claw his way out of his bed. My heart broke as I shut the door on my child. That night Gracin cried loud and hard for most of the night with small periods of a faint wine, which tortured my soul more than the tears. Although, in the morning, he moved with the same happy heightened alertness and did not seem to mind the lack of sleep. He did not hold what had happened the night before against me as I had envisioned. I was grateful.

The following night was by far the worst because he knew what was coming. He fought me from the time I took him upstairs, and he made his disapproval well known. He screamed with an ear piercing intensity during the night while I did my best to reread the pages of Dr. Weissbluth's book between my own shedding of tears. He went an entire night again without any sleep, and I was distraught.

The next day Gracin seemed to be somewhat worn out as he collapsed on my chest after breakfast for a ten minute nap. Looking down at my little boy sleeping, I did not know how much longer we could both go on like this. I felt I needed to be consistent with my choices, but I did not know how much more I could go through. I vowed to give this one more night before I would resonate to our old ways, but something amazing happened.

On the third night, with one final attempt at this method, after I had rocked and fed him, I placed my whimpering child into his crib. Turing to leave the room, Gracin pulled my arm and said, "I loves you Mamas. I dos." To my surprise after he said his part, he just laid there motionless until I walked out of the room. All that could be heard from his room was a faint whimper for the next five minutes. With the monitor's volume turned up, I watched as he thrashed his body back and forth, fighting with his mind to allow him to rest. Following the whimpering stage, there was fifteen minutes of faint crying, but then there was silence. That silence continued for the next eleven hours straight. I was amazed and ever thankful for the gift of sleep.

I felt my prayers had been answered when I awakened on the couch the next morning to light coming through the windows. In a slightly panicked state, I checked on the monitor thinking something had happened to my sleeping child. As I adjusted the contrast to see his perfect sleeping body, I heard the sweetest humming noise coming from his lips. He was singing to himself, and as he began to fully wake up, I watched him stand up and call for me.

In three nights he had figured out how to self soothe, and, as a result, I felt we had won our war on sleep. Our whole world seemed to open up. We saw that sleep helped Gracin calm down a little bit. It was ultimately what his body craved so deeply. After those first few nights, he still loved me all the more, but he actually asked to go to bed when he was tired. Of course, I cannot honestly say that Dr. Weissbluth's book fixed all of Gracin's sleep issues, but this was a step in the right direction.

Chapter 8: Rest, Peace, and the Correlation of Love

Frankly, as much as I would love to say that the daytime naps followed in the same suit as nights, I honestly cannot. I was amazed to read that naps are entirely different than nighttime sleep. Dr. Weissbluth states that, "Night sleep, daytime sleep, and daytime wakefulness have rhythms that are partially independent of one another." He goes on to state that "healthy naps lead to optimal daytime alertness for learning - that is, naps adjust the alert/ drowsy control to just the right setting for optimal daytime arousal. Without naps, the child is too drowsy to learn well. Also, when chronically sleep-deprived, the fatigued child becomes fitfully fussy or hyper alert in order to fight sleep." The charts presented on daytime sleep in Dr. Weissbluth's book really hit a nerve when I saw that Gracin was not even on the low end of the curve. According to the doctor, children at his age should be sleeping between 1 and 3 hours for a daily nap or two naps roughly totaling the same amount until their 22nd month (Appendix A on The Necessity of Sleep).

Although he was now getting the recommended amount of night sleep, Gracin was coming in between 40 and 60 minutes of broken sleep throughout the day that was not the least bit restorative. In reading about sleep fragmentation, I believed that Gracin's sleep patterns were affecting his development. His body did not know how to stay asleep. It needed to be taught, just as it did at night. In learning all about sleep schedules and how needed they are for a young child, I knew our lives must drastically change for Gracin's health and development.

Initially, it was again hard to put my child in his bed after we had just rocked to a calm state while he nursed and prayed. Using the cues for day sleep suggested, we decided that an early lunch, followed by our rocking routine, would be the best time to produce a long restorative nap. So, immediately after our 11:30 lunch we headed off to bed for a nap.

We used a twenty minute rocking routine, while nursing, with singing prayers and then put him down to sleep. Gracin, aware of what was expected of him, protested the nap for weeks. Although, after the third week, it was only the waking up too early that was hard. He would wake up not fully rested after about 20 minutes. Following the advice of Dr. Weissbluth's book, we again allowed him to cry for up to an hour from when he had first been put to sleep. This was the hardest time for me as he would scream, "Mama I awake" over and over.

I blamed our household situation that he was such a light sleeper. I thought we just needed to block out the background noise throughout the house. He could not sleep with the windows open. He could not have the slightest thing out of the ordinary occur before or during his naptime, or he would awaken. Although, it was not an easy task with not having our own home yet and being subject to unintended visitors and noises we could not control. I knew we could not wait to implement a structured naptime. It would be two months until we moved into our home.

To our surprise, by his 17th month birthday, Gracin was finally napping one to two hours a day and sleeping a straight twelve hours at night. I felt like I was floating on a cloud and my child was finally at peace, at least while he slept. In wanting to believe that Gracin's sleep would therefore heal his constant movement, I was saddened to admit that it did not substantially work that way. With all due respect to the author of the book that helped my son's sleep, it did not examine any cases of children with possibly hidden special needs or diagnosed special needs.

As Gracin's age progressed, he only became more impulsive, less adaptable, and had an ever-decreasing attention span. I felt powerless at what I could do with a child whose activity level gained in intensity with each passing day. As a result, I was left to questioning what love even was. Love could not be purely a feeling, as I had always thought, or I would have not made it this far. Fuzzy warm feelings were diminished greatly from my mind for my child, and I even questioned the saying that "Being a parent is the hardest job you will ever love." I could relate that it was the hardest job, but I did not think this was love at all. I was embarrassed by my child, placed into the spotlight of all eyes out in public, and made to look like I had no idea what I was doing with my little one. The games got old and my happy, calm, loving tone with my child began to diminish along with my optimistic thoughts of the future.

We were, in retrospect, in a wonderful situation, with a restored house almost completed, brand new belongings on the way, and a wedding in the upcoming weeks. Yet, I felt empty. I loved my husband-to-be, and I knew I loved my child, but our lives I did not love. I craved a feeling of love inside my being, but I did not, no matter how hard I tried, feel love. I was choosing to love, but was that what it was supposed to be: a choice? It did not seem at all as wonderful as I had always pictured in raising my own baby.

One day while reading a book entitled *Love and Responsibility*, written by Karol Wojtyla who became Pope John Paul II, love began to make sense again. Even the title defined this lightly used word more: there is a responsibility for acting in love. He states that "Love is an activity, a deed which develops the existence of the person to its fullest." I was completely taken aback that everything I had believed about love was based on feelings not the activity or the decision for the betterment of another individual.

That statement explained everything to me. Of course I was not happy, and I was not going to feel happy given my current thought process. I needed to choose to accept that love was the correlation of the actions that I was freely choosing to give my child. I needed to redefine the terms in my own mind. Those choices, therefore, would allow us over time to find, discover, and peel away the layers hiding our son's increasing needs. Love may have not seemed like enough before, but the superficial love and peaceful life that I had envisioned at the start of my son's life was not near the true definition of a total and self-giving love.

This child did take more. His needs truly brought to the surface many emotions, including sadness and anger, but that was the realization of my own lacking, not my child's. I had to choose to truly love him, as well as my spouse, giving up everything that came into our path as a potential detriment to our survival. I was loving all along, having the courage to do what was needed for my child even though my feelings felt saddened by those actions. I was being courageous by standing for my child's utmost wellbeing. I had no idea I was being loving in my actions just because it "felt" and seemed hard. I had to accept that feelings can misguide a person, and, consequently, an individual will not always feel the same. A person cannot be guided by feelings alone. A person must also use logic and reason, which dwell in the mind over the feelings that can confuse the best of individuals in being a purely physiological process.

Part 3:
The Overly Social Child

Chapter 9:
The Blind Climb

Moments passed. It became increasingly more difficult to see as the weather changed in velocity. The wind whipped the sand amongst the misty drizzle, while the purple sunset dissipated into its vast ocean bed. During the time that my gaze was again lifted to the heavens above, I witnessed the first synchronous crack and rumble in the skies. My heart sank in realizing that I should have been more aware of the weather all along. Those ever increasing gusts were my signal that a stronger storm was headed in our direction. Looking down to head for cover with my child, I felt dismayed when he was nowhere to be found.

Frantically looking around into the pitch-black night, I realized I was alone on the beach as I called out into the darkness of the storm. My mind beat upon itself. I began to search with tears filling my eyes. Calling out into the wind, I could barely hear my own voice over the humming of the gusts. As I prayed, searched, and cried, I saw our lifeguard begin to approach us once again. Feeling relieved in his presence, I signaled for help, but I was distracted by something out of the corner of my eye.

Feeling my heart drop, I turned to see a wave containing my baby. I rushed to reach my little boy, and I cradled his cold body in

The Blind Climb

my arms. Brushing the sand from his eyes and mouth, I helplessly felt the ground shake just as the sky again rumbled around us. With the blackened clouds enveloping the skies over the waterfront, I knew we had to quickly find shelter. My heart and soul were in distress. I swayed his body back and forth pondering my next move.

With movement returning to the tiny, wet, and cold weight in my arms, the only thing I knew to do was run. Although, in attempting to move us away from the storm, I froze, while an enormous wave crashed down over our heads. Feeling as though the ocean was determined to sink us down into its depths again, I felt my child gently lifted from my arms. Crawling out of the massive ocean that was beginning to expand upon the desolate beach, I followed blindly into the darkness.

Tracing the disappearing set of footsteps pushed into the sand, I felt I could not keep up as each step took more effort than the last. I stumbled clumsily back to the ground, landing with a large splash as the waves crashed again around me. Finally, getting unsteadily to my feet, I forced my body through the rising waters that had already reached above my knees. Just as I believed I could go no farther, dredging my body through the waves, I caught up to the lifeguard who was carrying my son. I paused to catch my breath and saw my child fighting to get down as the rain drenched his wispy curls.

With nowhere left to run or escape from the mounting waters, we raised our eyes to the unending abyss of a shadowy protrusion before us. The flashing night sky lit up our only way out. I felt hopeless. The top of the monstrous rock was not the least bit visible. Were we to free climb at an upward angle? Accepting our inevitable destiny if we stayed in our current place, we knew what we had to do. We could not let the surging waters drown us where we stood, no matter how hard our task at hand seemed. Trying our best to reason with a toddler who just wanted to dance in the storm, I ignored his protests, planted him on my back, and firmly placed my shaking grip on the first swelling of the cliff.

♥

Neuro-typical children, or those without an Autism diagnosis, are not robots. Although, things fall into place relatively smoothly with a good discipline strategy and consistency. In contrast, a child with an impending diagnosis, such as Autism or ADHD, as well as many other neurologically diagnosed special needs, can present their parents with quite a challenge. A child with High Functioning Autism has a hard time in a variety of new and stimulating situations. In one instance, they can totally impress you with their sense of knowledge of the world around them. In other instances, such as socially, they seem very far behind. Autism Spectrum Disorder is so broad that no two Autistic children are exactly alike, and that is why there is such a broad spectrum.

At the age of two, we really had no idea that our child was Autistic. In believing he was only special and unique, as his own person, we expected him to adapt as a typical child would. We broke routine, skipped some naps, and did what we wanted to do or felt would be fun for our child. We wanted him to fit into our lives, and we did not feel that we needed to change our patterns to fit into what he needed. How could he need anything else other than to be with his family?

We met with a doctor at every point suggested in his young life. Each time we received the same response: he was developing as a "normal" child should. In particular, at his 18-month visit, we were told that he did not have any signs of Autism because of how well he was able to communicate and have eye contact. He had met every milestone on time, if not early, but I still did not feel assured that he was developing typically.

Though, who was I to argue with a doctor who had years of experience? I was only a first time mom, young, and inexperienced. Now, looking back, I was the best person to stand up and fight for her child. I am so glad I did not accept what I was told and continued to push for answers, despite the naysayers, because it is by my research and my undying love for my child, that we were able to peel away the layers to his complex personality. What we revealed was something spectacular: buried beneath the behaviors was a little boy who truly wanted to listen, desired to show love, empathy, and the like, but he simply had no idea how.

Our complex two-year-old child was not the least bit typical in his actions. He moved like a hurricane destroying everything in his path, even though I do not believe he wanted to do that at all. Subsequently, I watched as the rising waters in his behaviors attempted to pull us under. I could not pass his actions off as the norm any longer. The wind, being his hyperactivity, only increased in momentum as he aged, and his constant talking became like a torrential downpour soaking us to our bones. As enlightenment came and we were led to accept, he was as overwhelmed as we were by his actions.

With each day that passed, we were ultimately pulling our bodies through what felt like a vast ocean. Frantically, we began looking for our way out. His impulsive bursts of unpredictability and at its height, violently expressed energy flashed erratically around us. With no idea where else to turn, staring at our little boy who had no idea what to do with all of his energy and movement, I contacted as many sources as I could to evaluate our son in his totality. We could no longer fight a battle through these undiagnosed symptoms on our own. Even though we were about to be informed of his "neurological diagnosis," we came to see the battle had not even begun.

Chapter 10:
A Mounting Paradox

I love my child. I love him more than I have ever known of love. Gracin has ultimately brought me to understand what it means to love; although, that fact in itself did not mean I could not be entirely overwhelmed by his behaviors. At the beginning, a mother's reason for being is to love a sleeping, movement-free addition to our world. That sleep reminds the parent of the good, the love, the work, the truth, that what they are doing day in and day out, moment-to-moment, has all been worth it.

The ultimate question, then, is worth what? What are we doing anyway as parents? Why are we raising these children who cause us so much stress after all? Are we doing it out of our own needs and the picturesque societal perfect family? Is there a white picket fence surrounding a large house with two perfect little additions playing in our back yard? Is our house big enough for our family of four? Do we get to go on fun trips multiple times a year? Do we make our neighbors jealous of what we have? Do we have just the right balance of happy and sad, wrong and right, to make us feel happy? Is everything perfect and new and shiny?

No, No, and most certainly no in our case. You see, I was nowhere near perfect, new, shiny, or where I thought I wanted to be as the days of my wedding approached. I never did desire to have what society stated as desirable. I had much larger, or in reality smaller, plans in my own mind. I wanted a large family with many children, as many as I was given, and although I craved to have a large house on a cul-de-sac in a nice neighborhood, all I truly wanted, at the root of my soul, was a peace-filled life in raising my family and the ability to enjoy their presence. I desired to be as Mother Teresa stated: "The Sunshine of God's Love;…God's Good News;…(and) God's Love in Action."

Yet, in our lives, with only one child, I was the opposite of that which I desired to be. Out in public I wanted to show others our happy and peace-filled life. Yet, to be as Mother Teresa stated, "Each time people come into contact with us, they must become different and better people because of having met us… We must radiate God's love," seemed impossibly out of reach with the child I had. I only had the desire buried deep inside to be real, calm, disciplined, and true to myself in all of my thoughts and actions. Though, in reality, I was horrible at showing the world what I was trying to be. By attempting to fit into the societal norm as well as act in the virtues stated above, I was ultimately failing at both.

Knowing that in only a few days I was about to marry a man who exemplified everything I ever desired in my heart, I had to make a choice. A choice away from what everyone knew me to be, or thought of me to be, into the person who I wanted to become. It was no longer about my desire, but a desire towards the future of our family and what we wanted to be known as, as a family unit. Even though I, myself, was greatly lacking in a multitude of areas, I knew that with our vows we would become one within the eyes of God. That was going to be my new start.

While my husband and I were starting off our marriage with a child, we really had little idea how much impact this would bestow upon our lives. After all, this child was not a calm, peaceful, little toddler. He, in his own right, was impulsive, ever moving, and complicated. This was, nevertheless, a result of my own decisions; therefore, the impact that this child bestowed on our life, by his developing ways, was no fault other than my own. Gracin was, in fact, the small puzzle piece of my life that I was trying my best to push into place. I did not have the time or the energy to deal with this challenge. I wanted and expected him to follow happily behind me like a duckling following behind his busy mommy. Well, of course, he wasn't a little duckling after all; consequently, there would be no following. He was, in fact, running full speed ahead of his busy mommy, as she had to change her direction to save him from many almost disastrous experiences.

Gracin, as I have stated, had many impulsive tendencies, but the scariest of all was that of the road. He had an intense obsession with the road. He desired to stand in the middle of each and every road and laugh with joy, but it was not funny at all. I cannot count how many times I scooped him up as a car slowed down for us or pulled him back as I collapsed into tears. He just thought it was so much fun, and that was about the extent of his play as we began moving into our new home.

Since toys were apparently boring, and the road was the best thing ever, Gracin would stand on the windowsills and stare at the cars passing by on that magical road of his. He would attempt to happily scream louder than the sounds made by the vehicles. Even though this was a very loud and questionable behavior, we did not think much of it. At the time, we just thought it was because he wanted to be outside and was being tormented by the passing of the cars. Since we were not inside with our little fireball all that much, the battle of wills between the cars and him inside did not seem to be of much importance. Although, when we were outside, he attempted almost constantly to be in the middle of his best friend - the road - and that made me extremely uneasy. I could distract him slightly by being in the backyard, but with the sounds of a passing car coming every few moments, my distractions were essentially useless.

My utmost attention had to be on my child. If I, for one split second, took my eyes off of him, to say hello to a passing neighbor or to answer the phone, he was like a rocket released to the road. The road was just too enticing for his mind. In addition, when he was outside and an ambulance, or "noisy car" as Gracin would say, began to approach, he would again dart for the road screaming as loud as he could while subsequently covering his ears. We believed he thought the road was the perfect place to scream with joy.

As a result, he made me look like the worst parent ever because who on this earth lets their child play in the road for fun as I seemed to do? The many glares, glances, and, at times, pep talks from strangers, were embarrassing. It was a horrific game that we believed he thought was of the utmost enjoyment, but in reality he was not acting out of enjoyment at all. We also thought he may be acting out of defiance and were dealing with a discipline issue. Although, as we came to see, he was only trying his best to show us his sensitivities. The almost constant rush of the cars passing and the noise and intrusion it was interjecting into his mind were actually hurting his head. He was only attempting to stop the noise by running into the middle of the road. His happy scream was his own way of drowning out the sound inside his head. Sadly, we had no idea at the time. We were as lost as we could be as to why he was doing these behaviors. We just wanted them to stop.

This little boy was pushing me to my limits, and he was barely two. We believed he thought everything was a game. It seemed

A Mounting Paradox

that every disciplinary direction that we gave him just made him laugh. It was horribly frustrating because he was so full of joy and smiles that it continued to make us wonder if he even understood anything that we were asking of him.

It is almost impossible to fully describe how much energy Gracin truly had. He could not sit still for seconds, let alone minutes, unless immersed in simultaneous rocking and prayer. It was like he was either on or off. There was no in between. He hated or loved something even for the smallest amount of time. Everything was completely and totally funny. It was funny if I cried at the side of the road at the thought of almost losing him to being hit by a car. It was funny if I got angry and smacked his butt for being in the middle of the road once again or screamed at him for doing something for the fifteenth time. It was even funny if I laughed at something cute he was doing. Everything was hysterical. Not one thing would faze this child, and nothing I tried would make him listen. No matter what type of punishment we used on him, it was a complete joke. He did not respond to redirection, time outs, a smack on the butt, or anything. We were at a total loss as to what to do.

No matter how much we watched him, his impulsive bursts landed him in some serious close calls. By the grace of God, nothing left more than a scratch on his body. You see, our son had no desire to follow in our footsteps and hold our hand like other kids his age. Even though other children do pull away from their parents and want to control where they go next, it was the constancy and number of times that our child did all of these behaviors that I am describing.

Most children respond very well to facial cues, but when we frowned and gave a look of disapproval, Gracin would just keep doing whatever he was doing. It seemed as if he felt he was being praised. Smiling at him also made him continue what he was doing because he would feed off of approval and become even more active and mischievous than before. He ultimately could not control his own energy level, and, therefore, was a danger to himself. We did pay attention to each and every behavior and sensitivity, but it turned out to be more avoiding what was causing him pain instead of helping to ease the sensitivity.

Gracin and I moved into the house a few days prior to the wedding day. In an attempt to help him respond as easily as he possibly could, we put a great deal of energy into replicating his sleeping arrangement perfectly. Happily, the transition to his new room was flawless. I was eternally thankful. Keeping everything consistent worked perfectly.

We gave him the biggest bedroom in the back of the house because it was the farthest from the sounds of the road. We decorated his bedroom with dark blue room-darkening curtains taped to his walls so to not let any light enter. Behind the curtain rods, I even taped foam backing so that light could not escape. A noise machine was placed under his crib set to the white noise setting. I had a specific line drawn with a black marker at the perfect setting for him to not hear a sound from the trucks passing by or if I dropped something in the kitchen. Standing in his room with the door shut, you would not have known if it was night or day, it was that dark.

We made every preparation for our light sleeper to allow him to sleep the best he possibly could. I was extremely proud of where we had come from and where we were at that moment. Even though I had no idea why my son was so fussy, we just made adaptations to our lives as any loving parent would for their child. We were thrilled to now be a true family, united by our marriage, as my husband moved into the house in the days following our wedding. It was the three of us against the world. We had no idea that we would soon feel as if we had the world against us.

Chapter 11:
Becoming What I Always Envisioned

This world – humans and animals alike - all function on predictability whether we want to admit it or not. The seasons, the days, the nights, all react in time to the rotation of the earth that always spins at the same velocity each and every day, month, and year. Therefore, our lives would be completely thrown off balance if one day the earth did not turn in the correct direction, at the same speed, or if it abruptly stopped turning. In the same way, we, as a people and society, function better on a typical daily schedule than in chaos.

Our bodies and our minds are not meant to live in a chaotic state. Living too long that way weighs on the mind and does not do the body good. In our world, a schedule seems only for the "boring old people" who are too stuck in their ways. Yet, those "boring old people" are the ones who hold the wisdom of the world. Wisdom brings insight, and insight is found after enlightenment into what our bodies are ultimately meant to do.

Our bodies are meant to function with a consistent sleeping and waking schedule in order to perform at optimum capacity. It is our choice to tap into that potential. As a result, why do we not help our children early on in their lives to feel the security from a predictable schedule?

Thankfully, my mind was slowly being shown what needed to be done within our own lives, to no credit of my own. This was more than likely God's plan. As we settled into our routine as a new family, I lamented my return to nursing school upon the close of summer. I believed I had finally found my niche in this world in being a stay at home mom. After much consideration, I desired it to become permanent. I knew that our lives would become more quiet and peaceful than ever before because I saw that our child was benefiting immensely with me being home. Gracin was sleeping consistently throughout the night, and, although he still had a lot of extra energy, I saw that when he was home with no unexpected alterations to his day, he responded differently.

With each day that passed, I knew my daily presence in his life could help restore more of his calm, but I felt so weighted down because I was also convinced that I needed to help our family out financially. Before the start of the clinical portion of my nursing school, I only had one class on campus a semester. I had done the rest while my son was only footsteps away, in online classes. Now I was basically going to need to live at school for the next four semesters until I graduated. I felt as if I was failing at being a mother by being away from him even though other family members watched him.

Upon returning home from my first full week in classes, I was excited to spend some extended time with my little boy, but he did not even care to acknowledge my existence as he ran around me in circles. He was overstimulated by so much movement and the lack of predictability from his week. I felt disheartened in hearing about Gracin's activity level, his protests over his nap, the erratic movements he was currently making, and the ultimate change in my son after only a week of classes. I knew, in that moment, we could not continue on like this.

As I poured out everything to my husband that night after Gracin was in bed, I felt misplaced in my own mind. I knew deep down what the right decision was for my family, but I was scared, scared to admit that everything I had worked for in my potential career could end in a matter of seconds. My husband did not deny any of the things that I said to him. He also believed that Gracin needed me more than we needed the financial gain. We agreed that I could not devote the next two years of Gracin's life placing him in the care of others. That night we made the decision together, our first real family decision, that in order to give this child what he needed, I could not go to school at this point in my life. I would be a stay at home mom.

Since I no longer needed to support this child on my own, this decision was easier. If I had still been a single mom, stopping school would have not been an option. I felt so blessed to have a husband who wanted me to be able to devote all of my attention to my child. In that moment, I put full trust in my husband to take care of us financially. The rest I placed in God's hands. Even though many nights I struggled with my decision, it was purely out of my own fear for our financial future. I also knew it was the best thing for this child. My mind kept going back to what Mother Teresa stated once: "There are many people who can do big things, but there are very few people who will do the small things."

My main focus now was to give myself up for the child to whom I had already given birth. Consequently, in that same month, we found out we were expecting an addition to our family of three. We were elated with joy. With all the blessings before us, I began to put our priorities in order for the future and our growing family.

I already knew how imperative it was for our son to have a strictly kept sleeping schedule. As for the rest of our hours, our time was extremely unpredictable. We ate when we got hungry, went outside when we felt like it, and went somewhere if we did not know what else to do. This type of behavior was not benefiting Gracin at all. I saw his naps slowly dwindling from two hours at seventeen months to one hour at twenty months. I knew we needed to restructure our time; although, I had no idea how. At the same time, I wanted to begin potty-training, and I felt the two would go hand in hand (See Appendix B: Toilet Training).

Chapter 12:
Discovering Autism

As much as I wanted to believe my child was your typical two year old, he just was not, for many reasons. Honestly, the most disheartening reason was his inability to show love to others. This sounds obscure to state about a two year old, but it was true. He did not know how to show he loved a person. He had no preference over his parents to strangers. He hated to sit in close proximity to anyone, and he certainly did not want to be cuddled, kissed, or hugged as he progressed in age.

There was one exception to the rule that changed his entire personality, and that was when he got sick. It was very odd, but his whole personality evolved when he had a slight fever. This led to many discussions between my husband and me as to why he was calm and peacefully happy only when he was sick. Now I am not talking about sick like he could not get out of bed. He, thankfully, never got that kind of sick. It was just when he had a slight cold with fever just over 100, his whole personality changed.

When he was sick, his mind, as a result, was put to ease, and he could just be. He wanted to be curled in our arms and read books, roll a ball back and forth, and act as a calm child typically would. It was a very strange thing that baffled me and led me to question more what was going on with my little boy. How was it that only when he was sick, was he calm, sweet, polite, and communicating what he wanted to say respectfully?

I wanted to experience this calmness in my child when he was not sick. I did not, as a result, wish he were sick more often. I wanted to restore the calm he experienced while sick into my child all the time. I did not want to be ultimately frustrated and anxious with my child's every movement. I desired to adore his presence. He moved too much, and I needed answers. I was only a month away from having a second child, and I needed to know what was going on in my little boy's head.

Upon researching this strange occurrence on the internet, I stumbled across my first article that illuminated a light bulb in my head to the word autism.

> According to a finding over the past few decades, parents and clinicians have observed that the behaviors of children with autism spectrum disorders (ASD) tend to improve, sometimes rather dramatically, during a fever. Longer concentration spans, increased language production, improved eye contact and better overall relations with adults and peers have all been reported. In a study published today in the Journal of Pediatrics, researchers from the Kennedy Krieger Institute in Baltimore, Maryland confirmed, for the first time, parent and clinician reports that the behavior of children with ASD improves with fever. The study evaluated children with ASD during and after an episode of fever and found that fewer autistic-like behaviors were recorded for children with fever compared to controls (Source: Kennedy Krieger Institute).

It was not just in my imagination. Here it was in my hand: a study that explained all of the questions that I had for my son, and my Gracin fell into the results of the study's findings. My mind was immediately taken back to the initial conversation with Gracin's doctor at his 18th month checkup when we filled out the M-CHAT or the autism questionnaire. Talking over the results with the doctor, I felt reassured that we passed that one, but was my relief justified? Thinking back, I never felt compelled to talk to the doctor about his toe walking, obsession with loud noises, sensitivities, or anything of the like as we went through the appointment questions.

I felt deeply saddened thinking that maybe I should have talked the doctor's ear off about every minute detail that I thought was different about my child. How else would he have been best able to evaluate what I was telling him? I was so worried about his activity level and impulsiveness, while being impressed by his language skills, that I pushed his sensitivities out of the conversation. As a result, his doctor just reassured us that these behaviors were how boys were. Leaving the office that day, I felt comforted that we were doing everything in the correct manner for our child, and I just had to accept I did not have the calm child I had always envisioned.

Although now, in this moment, after reading the article I held in my hand, I felt that he possibly could have autism. I had only ever heard of autism as being a type of disorder where children do not speak or speak very little, but that was not our Gracin at all. As I looked into autism and ADHD late into the night when the house was silent, I was astounded at what I found. Autism existed on a very large scale that included low functioning and high functioning as well as everything in between. I read and I read and I continued to read until my eyes could not be held open any longer.

Waking up the next morning, I just chalked up my night of searching to my overly obsessed mind projecting a condition onto my child that he could not truly possess. Though as time passed, the term kept coming back into my viewpoint. In a brand new study printed in *Pediatrics*, Dr. Amir Miodovnik, a developmental pediatrician at Boston Children's Hospital, correlated something that I always questioned in my own mind and heart. I now feared that my son's ever moving impulsive tendencies were masking a deeper rooted disorder: autism. Dr. Miodovnik states that, " Parents who believe that a child younger than 5 has ADHD should take their child to a developmental pediatrician, rather than a family physician, to make sure that possible autism will not be overlooked."

It was, of course, to no fault of our family doctor that my son's symptoms were missed. We, as parents, should have pressed the issue more to explain the extent of the activity of our tiny child. We should have seen a more specialized doctor and not accepted that our little boy was functioning typically, when in our gut we knew something was unique about our toddler.

In the same study, an alarming finding states that, "Autism and ADHD are very different neurological conditions, but they share a number of symptoms, genetic factors and brain pathways." This article states exactly what we were seeing in our child, yet we were experiencing it four years earlier. So yes, it may have been my fault that we missed the signs, but even though I blamed myself, I truly could not.

I was exhausted by the behaviors of my child, but most parents talk of how their kids tire them out. I have always felt disheartened because I did not press the initial doctor more because most children did not feel the same way Gracin did with his sensitivities. I did not understand why Gracin did not enjoy playing with toys, why the wind made him scream, why he walked on his tip toes, or why I could never read an entire book to him. Those facts aside, I still adored my little boy. My Gracin, with the wispy blonde curls and mesmerizing green eyes that reminded me of my father's own eyes, which I always desired to have for myself. This child still was part of me, and I did not want to complain about him. I only desired at the deepest part of my being to enjoy him.

With winter being at its most brutal point, we were cooped up inside too much, and our child was not reacting well. It was as if he was a racket ball unleashed inside our home. It seemed he never stopped moving or talking. I could not understand how a little person who was so small in stature, could talk so much and so well. He was speaking in full sentences now at 2 ½ with a vocal tone that was different than a typical toddler's.

He spoke with authority and knowledge, and that, in itself, made you forget how young he truly was. I even had to keep reminding myself of his age on various occasions. As he talked, he would dance around and constantly had to be moving different limbs simultaneously. He always held a joyful smile with burning anticipation radiating from his wide-open eyes.

He continued to not play as a typical child would and found enjoyment in counting his objects while dancing around them or spinning them. His body would not allow him to slow down enough to focus on playing with toys, even if he fully desired to, so there was no point in owning any. All he found enjoyment in was turning on light switches and spinning rolls of tape.

In attempting to find something, anything, to hold his interest so I could get household chores done, I turned to television. Here was something that almost all children enjoy. Gracin could care less. I searched and searched, but could not find any shows that would hold his interest other than one: *Dora the Explorer*. It is a high-energy show that encourages movement and has repetition of words, sounds, music, and people. Although it was the only show that held his interest, we could not bear the aftereffect. The "break" it bestowed on our lives was outweighed by the overstimulation it caused.

There had to be another thing that could hold his interest other than that show, but I felt I was missing it. One evening while waiting for my husband to get home from work, I collapsed on the couch exhausted and frustrated. I had been encouraging Gracin to play with toys all day to no avail. Gracin ran to the window and positioned his ear up against the glass. He heard my husband coming down the street and started singing a song at the top of his lungs, the exact song that was coming from my husband's car. I could not hear the music, but Gracin could. Even after the car was turned off, Gracin continued to sing the song while jumping up and down on the windowsill to catch a sight of his Daddy. To our surprise, he recognized the flow and rhythms of complex musicians, and we had no idea the way this would play into our lives in the future.

Gracin did not, in fact, enjoy typical children's music for more than a few seconds, but he could sit and listen to an entire Mozart symphony with its complex rhythms like an adult. We had finally found something that would instill peace in our child and help him stay calm. This was the perfect thing to keep his mind focused. I assembled an iPod entirely for his enjoyment. I added Mozart, repetitive prayer, and music with complexity for his growing mind. At night, Gracin and his Daddy sat together sharing one earbud listening to music as they bonded. During the day, Gracin and I enjoyed listening to various composers together while encouraging his focus on play. Music with rhythms and calming tones were what his mind needed so desperately. It was in those types of songs that we saw his body change slightly in its movement as his mind was able to focus on something else other than utter chaos.

There were so many things going on in such a small time period in his world that we just did not know what to expect. We were only beginning to discover how calm of an atmosphere our child needed, and we had no idea how our voices and actions could be affecting our child. Gracin would have benefited immensely to grow up in a home 200 years ago with no noisy toys, no cars passing by, where everything was calm and relatively predictable. Although impossible to perform time travel for our son, we knew we had to change our world to instill that same calm into his life.

Since every toy we owned would be pulled out within five minutes of him awaking in the morning, I knew we had to make a change. Our child's brain could not handle a toy box filled with toys as it over stimulated his mind. The toy box was daunting. Toy boxes and toys with noise attached only overwhelmed our son. These toys were only pulled out, turned on, and left in a pile behind him, littering my floor as he walked on to the next thing. I had not even gotten breakfast ready and already I, myself, was over stimulated. How could he not be?

I could not figure this child out! I was at a complete loss being alone with him nine hours a day when my husband was at work, and I could not imagine how I would care for another child soon. I loved this dear little joyful smiling boy with every part of my being, but I could not go on like this. I was saddened because I could not even find happiness in playing with my own child because of his short attention span. One day, out of total frustration, I put away all the crayons, finger paint, Play-Doh, paint, and paper and felt awful. All the items that I always felt I could do with my little child, and all the thoughts of how I envisioned our lives, just soared out the window with my patience.

Later that day, in attempting to play with trains on the floor for what felt like the millionth time, I broke down and cried. I could not understand what was causing my child to not act as a child at all. How was it that things as simple as trucks passing by, bubbles, finger-paint, or lotion upset my child? Why was it that the things every child loved, Gracin despised?

The only two activities that he truly enjoyed were running and talking, although talking would have won every time. Since his vocabulary took off at such a young age, it was not long before he was talking constantly. He talked to himself, talked in his sleep, talked while he was doing everything. It felt like he vocalized every thought that popped into his head. It was as if he could not understand that some thoughts were not meant to be spoken.

I had never met a two year old who would interrupt and control a conversation quite like this. Yes, most children do not understand how and when to come into a conversation, but this was different. He would take over, and it no longer mattered what you were saying because he either said it for you or the person you were conversing with simply forgot that you were even talking in the first place. Gracin always wanted to know what you were saying and demanded it with his famous line: "What you saying?" This was not once in a while or a cute thing. This was day in and day out with every sentence. This little boy would rather be a part of an adult conversation than play with toys. There was no way that being attention-deprived was at the root of his behavior either because I was with him constantly, and all we did was spend time together. I was never the parent who ignored him to watch TV, talk on the phone, or be on the computer. Those things were off unless he was asleep. All waking hours were spent with my attention on him.

It did not matter if you tried to ignore him while you were talking either. He would just climb up your body to look into your eyes demanding your attention. This child had no social fear, and he was OVERLY social. How did I have a child who was so opposite of me? It took me years to figure out how to even enter into a conversation and feel like it was the appropriate time. I never wanted to offend other people and would have rather kept my mouth shut than do anything to step on anyone's toes.

My husband and I were incredibly frustrated. Most children are very good at blocking out their parents while playing with their toys. They do not care what their parents are talking about, and when the parent tries to engage them in a conversation, they give one word answers and continue their play without even looking up once. Not this child. What was going on?

Most children have huge imaginations that make childhood a wondrous time of pretend play with dolls or cars, and that is all that matters in their young life. Not Gracin. We could not even have the simplest of conversations, such as asking what time it was, without his input. It became quite a large problem for us. Little did we know it would continue well into our future. We tried our best to only talk to each other once he was in bed, but by doing this, we were not teaching him anything. At the same time, we did not want to give him the impression that we didn't like each other.

As time went on, he would interrupt just to say he had nothing to say. He would then pause and begin to stutter only because he was thinking of what he could say next without losing the battle. He had nothing to say; he just wanted to be the center of attention. He was and needed to be the center of everyone's world. We did not want to raise a child who thought he was the greatest gift to the world. We had to do something! This problem may even seem trivial to most individuals, and maybe we should have let it go, but we did not know for how long it should be ignored. Until he was five, starting school, and did not know how to let any other kids talk?

This was the time to lead by example and not get frustrated with our son for expressing himself, but the balance was difficult! We attempted to have him say "Excuse me" before he would speak, but he would just keep repeating it constantly during a conversation. To his credit, he was polite. It was just that he was not picking up on the cues of how often to speak. He did not understand the parameters and boundaries that most children pick up on very easily without instruction. He understood speech and could easily memorize what to say. He just did not get anything past the "coached" behaviors we taught him. It was as if he just said everything in his head because he had no idea about the next thing to say. We could not play, talk, eat, or interact the way we wanted him to, and my gut feeling that something was wrong just kept getting stronger.

I must say I felt more like an utter failure at being a mother than anything else on most days, but we were still having more good moments than bad at this point. Though as he got older, everything seemed to get more and more difficult. He began to move so much that his face would get flushed when we were only at our daily routine. Even though I would love to say that his sleep duration continued to be in the optimal range, that slowly diminished. For naps, even though he spent a quiet time in his bed in the afternoon, he was only sleeping two, maybe three, days per week, if we were lucky.

I learned to turn my phones off and unplug the doorbell. The house became so quiet you could hear a pin drop, and the slightest noise during a nap, such as a lawn mower or snowplow, made me cringe beyond belief. Even with a noise machine running to almost the highest degree in his room, a person still could not enter the room below him during his sleeping hours. I relied heavily on his video baby monitor in order to keep an almost constant eye on his napping routine.

Looking back on that time period of our lives, I truly felt that I did everything in my power to help Gracin grow. My days were spent giving him stability where he needed it most. I changed everything about how we acted day to day and moment to moment. We did everything for this tiny soul who I knew could grow up to make an impression on the world. At each day's end, we reflected on what we could do differently as parents to help our son and apologized for what I felt was done wrong. It seemed that our lives had just begun to bud, and, as we welcomed home our new addition to the family, we were elated with joy. Unfortunately, life did not stay on the upswing for long.

Comparably, nothing in my son's life was quite on the traumatic side, such as what happened a few months before his third birthday. Up until that point, he was really just a very busy child who never stopped moving. He had never before presented any violent tendencies or the like. He was kept relatively close to us and was always with a family member if we had to be away for any reason, which was not much. This moment in particular will never leave my mind. This was the point when I knew we needed real help, and we could not wait until he was in school as his doctor had suggested.

We had my grandparents over. As I was cleaning up from dinner, I noticed a drip coming from the ceiling. Since my grandfather was always the one to jump in and help in any situation, before I even turned around to tell my husband what was happening, my grandfather was on his way up the steps. As the moments unfolded, my husband was preoccupied with helping upstairs while I finished cleaning up, and Gracin was running back and forth in the living room in front of my grandmother who was holding the baby. Since I knew Gracin would not go to sleep with visitors in the house, I was not even going to bother trying to put him to bed until they left. I told Gracin he could watch a TV show until my grandfather was done fixing our plumbing issue. He was thrilled.

I still remember him, clear as day, climbing up so excitedly next to my grandmother to watch *Dora*. I took the baby from her arms, and Gracin grabbed his leg gently to kiss him before I put him to bed. I bent down and looked Gracin directly in the eyes. I explained that I was going to put his brother to bed, and he was expected to sit on the couch until I returned. My grandmother reassured me that he would be fine and to take my time. I felt comfortable for the most part with her watching him with me only footsteps away, but I was still skeptical. To this day, I wish I had NEVER left him alone with her.

Moments after walking up the stairs, our lives suddenly took a new turn. Our sweet little son, whom we thought was just hyper and filled with undrainable amounts of energy, did not seem so sweet anymore. I had just completed dressing the baby for bed when I saw my husband and grandfather beginning to go down the steps. I felt relief that my grandmother was only alone for moments with our rambunctious son. My relief did not last long, though, as I heard my husband run the remainder of the way down the steps. I immediately felt sick to my stomach as I also ran downstairs to see my husband ripping Gracin off of the couch. I had never seen him as upset as he was that night. Gracin was standing on the couch kicking my grandmother in the chest repeatedly while she begged him to stop.

I had only been upstairs for five minutes at the most, and he had done this! I was so worried about my grandmother that I really paid no attention to anything else. She reassured us that she was absolutely fine and kept saying that Gracin was just trying to play with her, and he did not mean it. I had a hard time justifying the behavior. As we placed him in time out, they voiced their disapproval in how we were handling the situation. They were defending a child who had just kicked an older woman at least three times in the chest. What type of parents would we be if we did not punish him for his behavior? He was going to be in time out, and there was just no way around it.

Before they left, we had him apologize to my grandmother. When he was asked why he chose to do something like that, he responded with a smile, saying he just wanted to. How could this child look at us straight in the face and say with a smile that he just wanted to kick someone in the chest. He thought it was funny, amusing, a game. We needed help, fast. I knew that this child was not just hyper. Something physiological was going on. We could not and we would not let this type of behavior slide. I was going to do everything in my power to make sure that this child would never hurt anyone again. I had already been very limited in the times that I had been away from his side, but now everything had changed.

The next morning I made the first phone call to start our journey in helping our son to a developmental pediatrician. In my opinion, my sweet little boy was gone, and, sadly, I now looked at him as a potential danger to everyone around him. I would not walk out of the room anymore without him by my side. I would not trust him alone with himself while I went to the bathroom for a moment. I felt that I couldn't even trust him around anyone in the family. We were appalled at his behavior, and we could not understand it at all.

We received criticism from some that he was just a kid, and kids do stupid things. However, I was not going to let him hurt anyone - no matter who they were. It seems trivial, but I had to do something to express my anger towards him, so I cut his hair. I remember feeling anger that I had never felt before radiate throughout my bones as I snipped the baby curls off his neck. He was not acting like a sweet little boy anymore, so he did not deserve these sweet little curls. It may sound harsh, but my baby had hurt one of the most meaningful and wonderful people in my life, and I was mad. I had never before shown him how mad I was, had never screamed at him or smacked him out of anger, but I needed to do something now. As I put ear buds in his ears and got out the shears, I shaved his hair down to nothing.

Watching those curls fall to the ground, I cried and cried. I may have cried because of what had happened, but I felt like it was because I had screwed up everything. I blamed myself, and as those pieces of hair fell, I looked at my life falling to pieces. I felt a great deal of regret. What did I do? Why did my son find joy in inflicting pain on others? What was I to do? Looking back, really I had nothing to cry at, but wrapped up in all of the emotion of his first violent episode, I only knew how to cry.

We know all too well that with life changing so rapidly it is easy to miss or ignore behaviors because they are inconvenient at the time, difficult to accept, or hard to explain. There are too many excuses, too much to do, and not enough time to work with our children in the demanding world in which we live. Most behaviors are ignored and pushed aside until one happens that can no longer be ignored, as we experienced. We had convinced ourselves that he was just bored with only an adult as a playmate. As he aged, we thought his attention span would increase, but we were wrong.

There was something else going on in his mind that needed a heightened level of attention. I was now forced to no longer ignore his "quirks." I could not be blinded by a parent's love for her child and not admit that something was different in his developing mind. I had to use the love of his soul, the love of his person, the love I did not feel- though knew I possessed - in those passing moments to push through the anger and give him what he truly needed. He needed help for his mind. Yes, he could still have prayers and be given love. Though what he needed more, at that current moment, was not what typical children need. Gracin needed something more.

Part 4:
Not One, but Three Diagnoses

Chapter 13:
A Violent Shaking

The rock shook with a multiple of thunderous rumbles before I had even mustered the courage to bring my entire body to the base. As I stood there, with the rising waters engulfing my legs, I questioned if I, myself, encompassed enough strength to endure this next trial. With hundreds of questions filling my mind, I became lost in trusting that I could successfully reach the summit on my own merit. I did not believe that I could do what I felt I had to do, yet I believed I had no options left. Repositioning the heavy and thrashing child on my back, I begged him to hold on as I swallowed hard and simultaneously pulled my drenched legs out of the water.

In finding each small ledge for my footing, I could only pray that my next movement would not cause me to slip down into the freezing waters. I was forced to dig my nails into the cliff for support as the entire rock again began to shake with the roar of the thunder echoing throughout the vicinity. As the sun disappeared entirely, we were left in complete darkness. With no visual idea of where I was climbing, my only physical guide was the rock that held my cold and shaking body. The dropping temperature made

A Violent Shaking

the arduous climb close to impossible, but nothing could now deter my mind from what needed to be done.

I felt my body breaking down with each change in position; however, I was determined to hold on for the life of my child. There was no relief. My hands cracked and became numb, while, at the same time, my back tightened and ached from the weight upon my shoulders. My body became bruised while scaling the jagged cliff side as we were slammed into it by the force of the gusts. It seemed as though not even the wind had an intention on providing us with any type of relief as every element in our vicinity seemed determined to have us fall. With tears streaming down my cheeks, I silently begged for some type of a rest.

I was so worn down by the climb that I felt despair set in as to if we would ever make it to the top. With yet another flash of lightning, I looked up searching for some view of what lie ahead. All I saw was rock. The rain continued to burn my frozen face with each drop that felt as though needles were countlessly protruding into my skin. I could truly not move one more muscle, and in one split second, my body shut down in its place.

I felt trapped, scared, and out of breath as I began to believe this climb was in fact impossible. There was no longer any strength left in my body. I knew I could no longer do any of this on my own. I had put much belief into my own abilities, even though I knew that I was, after all, just one human being who encompassed really nothing on her own. I was not fit to lead a climb, make decisions, or any of the like, but it was in that moment that I knew exactly who could.

In attempting to regain my strength once again, I bargained with my child to hold on for just a minute longer, while I rested in place. Though, to my surprise, just as I began to close my eyes, my glimpse found a ledge of significant size to the right of my body.

Reaching for that ledge with all of my strength, I pushed my child up to safety first. As I hoisted myself up, I collapsed entirely in tears. I sat down holding my child tightly on my lap, kissing his forehead before feeling the embrace of our lifeguard from behind.

As we sat in safety for just a few moments, we stared out into the black nothingness of the sea. I could not do much other than thank God for the ability to rest during our arduous journey and promise that I would now rely on Him as my ultimate guide. I was so thankful to again be able to hold the dear little child whom had now fallen asleep beside me. In that moment, I also attempted to sleep, but sleep eluded me. I was incapable of resting when I knew that at any moment my child might try to escape our position. With the two bodies sleeping beside me, I reclined against the rough wall as I again stared out into the darkness that surrounded us. When the sky flashed, I was able to peer into the heart of the storm. My weighted eyes eventually fell closed, just for a brief moment. Against my own will, I was immediately taken into a sleeping state.

Awakening only what felt like seconds later, the sun had begun to rise. I could now vividly see the devastation the hurricane had bestowed upon the beach. Gazing into nothing but ocean, I watched as the rain from the skies above surrounded the base of the cliff. The beach was entirely gone, and the waves pounded upon the rocks below. The wind continued to whip and howl, while far out in the distance, I could vaguely see some calm waters. Seeing calm on the horizon, I became invigorated with hidden energy as I fully awoke determined to finish our climb.

I looked beside me and watched as my son joyfully sat with our lifeguard throwing tiny pebbles into the massive sea below. Smiling happily at the sight of them, I felt reassured that we were doing the correct thing in climbing with a newfound devotion to

A Violent Shaking

who was really in control of our lives. As we began to prepare to climb once again, my son protested loudly with endless screams while I held onto his small body. Attempting to thrash loose from my grip once again, I reassured him with calm and firm words as I began to scale the wall. Simultaneously, I began praying deep within my own soul for strength. Even though the rain still poured down from above, our mission did not seem as devastating as before because we now held the faith to push onward.

♥

With the battle of a lifetime before me and my family, I was led to question everything in its complete totality. I believe every life has a point where a person hits a sort of bottom and realizes just how little they truly are in the grand scheme of things. I, personally, believe that I have hit that low point countless times, but one of the longest, lowest, periods of my existence was during my oldest son's 3rd year. There was entirely too much of everything going on, and silence itself seemed a fairytale. I had never felt more worn down than that year with my child; at the same time, I believe that it was just as hard for him.

I was determined to give this child every part of my body and soul, yet even that seemed like not enough. My desires, overpowered by my exhaustion and my own anger at the situation, seemed to get the best of me. I could not control my son's violent hour long meltdowns, which brought me to my knees. I could do nothing to help the screaming. Even my touch made him only scream louder. He did not want any sort of physical affection at any point throughout the day or night, and during these outbursts, that at their height occurred five times a day, my mind was left in complete shambles. I did not understand how holding him brought out a violent and intense anger in his eyes that a parent should never have to see in their little child.

I did not believe that I was doing anything correctly. Although, looking back, I see that my husband and I did exactly what needed to be done. We did not force our love on our child in the manner we believed he should be loved. We gave him the appropriate outlets to express his own anger, while we, at the same time, gave him tools to calm his own mind. We did not leave the house for that full year with him unless we had to go to a doctor appointment or something of dire need. We did not go grocery shopping together, go out in public, break routine, or anything of the like because our son needed the stability, consistency, and predictability of knowing what would happen next in his life.

We basically sheltered ourselves in an attempt to regain control over Gracin's emotions in order to allow his body the stability it craved. We hoped we could then slowly incorporate in new situations without meltdowns. We did a complete turnaround between the ages of two and three, where instead of expecting our son to fit into our lives, we now sacrificed ourselves for our son's ultimate wellbeing. It was hard, no close to impossible, yet it was exactly what love calls us as parents to do.

Our love was enough. It was enough to climb up any rock without a guide into the heart of the storm. With the sight of our son's soul in mind, I abandoned every thought of myself for his wellbeing and gave him every ounce of my body in service to his good. It may seem as if we trusted too much in our own devices, yet I personally feel that we did not trust in ourselves at all. We trusted in God that He would bring us into the sunlight once again. We trusted in prayer, good works, and perseverance to keep us safe and straight on our arduous climb.

Of course, I was not alone on my journey as God had blessed me with an exceptional husband to help when I believed I could do no more. I felt as though I was blindly feeling my way, yet by using my faith to stay true to my son's needs, I was never fully in the dark. To my disbelief, all of our perseverance to find out answers for our son led us to the correct doctors who properly diagnosed him.

After encountering numerous doctors along our way, we were given our much needed rest as we watched our son sleep deeply and actually play with toys for a substantial period for the first time in his life. As we rested on what felt like a ledge high above the raging waters, we were not only given our son's diagnoses, but we were also given peace of mind. The diagnoses were hard to swallow yet made sense and helped us to give our son's mind the exact kind of calm that his body always craved. The two neurological diagnoses of High Functioning Autism, also known as Asperger's, and ADHD gave us a direction and an illumination to push onward. At the same time, our son's behavioral disorder, termed Intermittent Explosive Disorder, was brought to light as we attempted to find ways to best help his mind find a calm way to express emotions. As a result, we were led onward towards the future, a bright future where our son excelled at life instead of being overwhelmed by it.

Chapter 14:
Our Reset Button

Gazing deeply into those large, green, and wide-open eyes at 3 o clock in the morning for what felt like the millionth night in a row, I once again questioned everything. My mind encircled itself as I begged my child to close his eyes once again to allow his body to fall back to sleep. Yet, all I heard countless nights in a row was, "I not tired Mommy," "I already slept," or "I don't know how to close my eyes." My attempts at explaining that two, four, and six hours of sleep were not enough rejuvenation for a tiny body were close to useless. To no avail, a few hours later the process would again be repeated. As my husband and I rotated the sleep routines, we became just plain exhausted. Our youngest son, at this point, was sleeping peacefully twelve hours throughout the night, yet it seemed that there was no end on the horizon for our Gracin's sleep habits improving. Gracin truly believed he was not tired. What bothered me almost as much as the loss of sleep was how our child could not understand how to close his own eyes. We could not understand how he honestly did not know how to do this, yet we had no idea how to help him. We all were at a heightened breaking point as the dark circles under his eyes were in fact becoming black dark bags.

Gracin's brain would not allow his body to rest in this current situation, and we ultimately were discouraged for the future. I felt as though my son, and we as his parents, were being tortured. I had heard of children who woke in the middle of the night to go to the bathroom, because they had a nightmare, or wanted to sleep with their parents, but a three year old who desired to sleep in two hour sleep/wake intervals was unheard of in my mind. Exhaustion loomed over all of our heads, but, somehow, the only one who seemed to be unaffected by it was our son! In fact, he seemed to receive more energy with the less sleep he got.

I felt as if I was failing him as a mother. I practiced having him close his eyes during our daily routine but quickly became convinced he truly had no idea what closing his eyes meant. On top of that, he did not even understand many of the facial expressions that I asked of him, such as smiling, making an angry face, and the like. I was not only lacking in energy from the situation, but I also felt as though a wedge was placed between my child and myself. I could not understand why touching Gracin's hair, rubbing his back, or picking him up made him so tense. I felt as though I could do nothing right for his person, even though I wanted my loving embrace to be enough to fix his entire world. I prayed, oh how hard I prayed. Yet, I felt, at the time, that I was receiving no answers.

I knew that I could not just sit around praying for a miracle, even though a miracle to heal all of his sensitivities was what I wished for more than anything. Something had to be done. We could not live like this, scratch that, we refused to live like this any longer. The stress was pervasive, and I could no longer subject our family to this pain day in and day out. We had to get some answers, but really, was a psychiatrist our solution?

Our Reset Button

I felt so torn! I wanted a reset button, a large red magical button that would restart our lives yet still provide us with the knowledge we had gained these past three years. Unfortunately, that button did not exist. Although, resetting our lives while remaining at our current point was, in fact, the best course of action.

As strong as I attempted to be, I slowly began to be worn down by my own lack of sleep. When I caught sight of myself in the mirror - that I can promise you I avoided like the plague - I would become sullen. I saw my own dark circles, and I felt as if I was aging greatly by the minute. If it had not been for my husband's loving devotion, I may have sunk into a deep depression because I began to have thoughts of horrid proportions creep into my mind. My husband was my stronghold, my rock, and my stabilization. He guided me to seek comfort in God instead of the earthly comforts I felt myself seeking. It was difficult, yet I began to find solace in reading small chapters out of the Bible in those long dark days. One of my favorite quotes on life's struggles is from 1 Corinthians 10:13 where it states that, "No trial has come to you but what is human. God is faithful and will not let you be tried beyond your strength; but with the trial he will also provide a way out, so that you may be able to bear it."

As I read chapter by chapter of the Bible, I became convinced that the man who I married was not just the man with whom I chose to spend my life. I truly believed he was also placed on my path as the way out of my old life, help with raising my Gracin, and finding the correct path for myself in relying fully on Christ. Yes, I was being tested in the darkest hours of the night when my will was at its lowest points, and I was more readily to snap. This, though, was just another trial I had to bear. This trial led us to find ways to help this child, whom to us was gifted, to find the techniques to reset his own mind. As God was my way out, I was my son's way through this life to his eternal destination. We knew that his life was not going to be easy for him or us. It seems to be, that in this life, the largest struggles sometimes produce the strongest people.

I felt as if we were hitting our lowest points in order to lead us into acknowledging that we really did need the specialist. We never wanted to be the parents who gave their child medication, but everything was brought into question at this time. As we resolved to at least meet with a specialist, I gave up everything that did not need to be done. Consequently, we truly functioned in basic survival mode.

I cared for my children during the day, read bits and pieces when I could, slept almost every moment that my children did, and the rest of life just had to wait. I developed a very basic schedule for our household duties, and if I could not do what needed to be done for that day, my husband took over after he got home from work. We ultimately relied on each other to pick up where the other one could not.

Our nights dragged on slowly and seemed to never end. Our days, frankly, were not much better. I could think of nothing to keep Gracin occupied. It was an awful feeling to have a house full of toys with not one toy being played with by him for more than a few moments at any given time. He had no interest in typical children's toys; although, he was rarely seen without his tape roll in hand or standing at a light switch. These facts seemed to show us that he could hold sustained interest in certain types of items, but we could not understand his fascination with his chosen items. I did not fathom his obsession with spinning objects or the control over the light switch, but I attempted to find ways to have growth within his preoccupations.

Our Reset Button

In a basic attempt to help him slow his bodily movements and actions down, I began counting out everything for Gracin. We counted steps we took, pushes on the swing for his baby brother, laps he ran around our yard, times the tape roll spun, and anything else I could think of. After seeing how incredibly easily he learned counting, we purchased Gracin his first watch.

Who would have thought a watch, such a common thing for adults, would bring such enjoyment to a small child. His first digital watch literally never left his wrist, and since he was already able to count to at least one hundred while recognizing most of those numbers, his watch helped him understand what time it was. As a result, he was then able to know when he awoke in the middle of the night, if he could now get out of bed, or if he needed to go back to sleep. The watch helped us immensely because it was the reminder his little brain needed to have some control over his world.

At the same time, he was in the process of discovering how to get out of his crib, so we had yet another transition ahead of us. Thankfully, I found a lifesaver called, My Tot Clock and this alone made the transition from crib to toddler bed quite close to flawless. Within a few hours, I was able to roughly teach Gracin how to read not only the color coding system of the My Tot Clock but also how to read the hand directional of the analog design. This clock is so amazing that I think all young children should have one. My Tot Clock gave Gracin something to listen to and focus on as he drifted off to sleep, so he was not lying silently in the dark after we said our good nights. The clock's blue and yellow lights let him know when it was okay to get up (yellow) and when it was still quiet or nighttime (blue). It also read him a bedtime story, played music, and gave white noise all throughout the night. Honestly, I wanted to give the inventor a hug when we received it since we saw immediate improvement in our son's sleeping habits.

Even though we were seeing these gains in his nighttime sleep, we knew we could do more to help Gracin sleep more continually throughout the night. He was still only sleeping in two-hour increments, and lying there awake during the night while we slept, even though he was quiet, scared me more than anything. We discussed putting a lock on the outside of his door to keep him safe in his room, but I knew there had to be a better answer. I was frankly scared to sleep even though sleep was what my body craved most.

After reading Dr. Weissbluth's book once again, we decided to implement an extremely early bedtime to reset Gracin's internal clock. As I read, a light bulb illuminated in my own mind as the following words brought comfort to my overwhelmed thinking: "Try a temporarily super-early bedtime to help him wake up better rested…Often, the early bedtime will help erase his sleep debt so he is more able to relax." The book only advised this for a child under three years of age, but we felt we had to try anything to help our child sleep better, both at naps and continually throughout the night. Although it sounds harsh, it WORKED. Even though this method was aimed mainly at reestablishing an afternoon nap routine, we saw positive night sleep benefits as well. In addition, we also got a big dry erase board, as suggested by the doctor, tweaking the "Sleep Rules" from his book to our own liking. We also moved Gracin's bed into a room that directly led to a bathroom so that he could go to the bathroom without needing our help in the middle of the night. The following are the rules that we developed for Gracin's sleep:

1. Lie down
2. Stay quiet

3. No kicking or yelling
4. Close your eyes
5. Go to sleep
6. Do not get out of your bed unless you have to use the bathroom (only 1 time)
7. Half an hour show or game if you follow all your rules
8. We will watch you on the monitor and keep you safe
9. Mommy and Daddy love you
10. God is also going to watch over you to protect you and keep you safe

After all of the changes were in place, we began to implement his new routine the following day. After dinner, I turned all the lights in the house down to a slight dim. We had a half an hour prayer time combined with rocking, and then it was right to bed at no later than 5:00 p.m. We did this for two weeks. Then gradually, using the clock, the rules, and lots of reminders, the bags under Gracin's eyes significantly diminished. We were amazed with how much improvement came from an earlier bedtime.

Because Gracin was still waking up in the middle of the night two to three times, he was given a rosary, and we encouraged him to pray himself back to sleep without our intervention. Naps even improved. He was quieter and calmer and napped three to four times per week for an hour, which was a huge gain for us. After three weeks, we delayed his bedtime by ten minutes each night until we started seeing it affect his sleeping pattern. We concluded that he slept the best from 6:00 until 10:00 p.m., and since we were not willing to sacrifice those four straight hours of sleep, we kept his bedtime at 6:00 p.m. Most of his third year he went to bed at 6:00 p.m. He continued to nap at least three days per week and continued to have a quiet time daily from 12:00 -3:00 p.m. since we never knew at what time he would allow his body to sleep. This quiet recharge time was good for his mind as he learned to rest, pray, and establish a time to be with only himself. During that time, he was without any outside stimulus. He had no intrusions into his world such as the phone, doorbell, cars passing by, or the unexpected. I learned to make the house silent for him during those times, and we were happy to see how much he benefited from being on such a predictable schedule.

He was better rested; his brain was better able to absorb information given to him, and his intellect just seemed to take off. Since I had no idea what to do with my vivacious ever-moving child during the days, I started to teach him a rough Kindergarten curriculum on my own. I quickly discovered that Gracin was already more advanced than I had ever given him credit for.

He had always astounded us with his intellect, yet I really never considered him more advanced than other children until the one moment that changed my outlook. One day, as I was finishing cleaning up from lunch and I saw Gracin's body dart past me after one of our cats, I quickly mentioned that he only had a few minutes left before naptime. Thinking no response would be coming, I turned to finished cleaning, but the response I received was jaw dropping. I still can picture the exact place in our house where I was standing and even what Gracin was wearing when he first stated, "I know Mommy. I have thirteen minutes left." As I turned to look at the clock on the stove, chills went down my spine in seeing that the time was 11:47 a.m. checking myself to make sure I was not imagining what I believed to be impossible, I walked over to my little boy. Glancing down at his watch to see the same time that was shown on our stove, I quickly bent down to ask Gracin how he knew that. My question, though, was too vague, and he ran off before I could say anything else. Catching my breath, I called my husband at work as I stood there shocked and in disbelief. My husband laughed and said something to the effect of it just being a lucky guess. Though that night, with multiple questions posed at our son, we saw it was more than a lucky guess. Gracin knew exactly how to tell time.

Within the days that followed our discovery, we moved on from numbers, to letters, and to putting letter sounds together. We did notice that it seemed he could go much further as he began to become angry when he already knew something that we were asking him to repeat once again. So we moved on to harder mini lessons such as memorizing sight words and ultimately learning to read. Gracin amazed us with his knowledge and his quickly advancing intellect. We were astounded at how easily learning just seemed to come to him. He, in effect, taught himself to read with only my guidance, but I cannot credit it to myself at all. His ability to memorize was flawless, and to this day, I wonder if he has a photographic memory. Although we could not connect through play, we had finally found something that would hold his interest for mere minutes, and we were pleased at that.

Chapter 15: Sensitivities, Frustration, and Finally Enlightenment

Finally, after what felt like years of waiting, we took our first step towards the answers we were seeking. I was so frustrated in the waiting game of the pediatric specialists that I attempted to find a way to get Gracin evaluated sooner in a roundabout way. My grandmother had suggested that certain food allergies may cause hyperactivity symptoms, so I thought an appointment with an allergist could not hurt.

 We arrived on time and had a twenty minute wait, which may have been expected for a busy doctor's office, but with each passing second, the stress mounted. Gracin was a ticking time bomb especially when confined to close quarters, and this busy child did not amuse his middle-aged audience. Gracin was always known to get everyone's attention, so when he began to see that his new "friends" were ignoring him, he tried all the harder to get their eyes on him by being destructive. I will admit that my child was memorable and caused everyone to notice him, but, unfortunately, this was not in a "look how cute he is" way.

 My child had no boundaries, and climbing onto a stranger's lap was just another fun thing to do to get them to look in his eyes, which were half an inch away from their faces. Though within a split second, he would be on to the next person's lap, and I, helplessly, had no control over him. I could only hold him in my arms for so long. Having him fight and scream that I was hurting him made me feel like absolutely the worst parent ever. I must have looked ridiculous to all of the spectators with my arms tightly wrapped around his little body as he tried to break free from my grasp. With every door that opened, a new pulse of energy would emanate throughout his body as he tried his hardest to break free of my grasp.

When our name was finally called, my eyes were welling up with tears out of complete embarrassment, exhaustion, and shame. Although, in reality, his behaviors were of no surprise to me. New situations changed my child into an over stimulated mess of a little boy. I felt awful that no matter how hard I tried, I could not control Gracin's actions or help him feel relaxed in new situations. I honestly believe that to an outsider I did not appear as the loving and devoted mother that I actually was. In my mind, I knew I had to be constantly aware of any possible scenario that may happen to pop into Gracin's head in order to be one step ahead of the game. Unfortunately, by being so constantly aware of my son, I seemed to be a stressed out over-protective parent. It was not by choice that I did not smile or make friendly chit-chat. I just couldn't. My brain would not allow me to think of anything but what my child was capable of doing next.

As Gracin pulled my tightly wound hand down the long hallway, I felt as if we were the laughing stock of the waiting room. While remaining in our examination room for another five to ten minutes, Gracin literally bounced off of the walls. When the allergist finally made his appearance, Gracin greeted him with the smartest comment that could pop out of his mouth, demanding to know how old the doctor was. After a small begrudging laugh, I

Sensitivities, Frustration, and Finally Enlightenment

attempted to explain our situation while having a child who interrupted just about every word that I said. Gracin's face was so close to the doctor's, he was practically touching him. I struggled with trying to get my words out and correcting my son at the same time, but, thankfully, this new doctor caught on quickly and started only asking questions that could be answered with a yes or no, which Gracin still attempted to answer for me.

The doctor ordered a standard allergy test, which unbeknownst to me did not test for any food allergies. This test was done by little pricks all over his back, and I was warned that most kids cry. Well, to the nurse's disbelief, my son just laughed hysterically with each prick. Everything was a game to him, so it did not really surprise me, but his pain tolerance was unbelievable. The allergy test came back negative to everything except one mold spore type, and I felt heartbroken. I wanted so badly for this to be our answer.

I believe the allergist saw my frustration as I continued to take an unreasonable amount of abuse from my son who made it known that he was more than ready to go home. As the doctor and I attempted to finish our conversation, in a final effort, he described to me a food diet called the Feingold Diet, which had been known to help children with ADHD. He told me that he could not be sure that ADHD was an accurate diagnosis, but he stated that he saw a food additive diet work wonders on children with various levels of hyperactivity. He also suggested that I take him to a pediatric specialist who could truly diagnose and treat Gracin because he felt that there was more than just ADHD to be concerned with. He gave us a number for a local psychiatrist, and I thanked him for all that he was able to do.

As we left the office that day, I felt hopeless. No diet was going to cure this child, but we had to try something. As I strapped Gracin into his car seat and attempted to quickly place the new number in my phone, I realized that we were already on that waiting list. A tear fell slowly down my check in the ultimate defeat. I could not stand to sit through another doctor's office wait like the one I just endured. I felt as if we wasted our entire day just to get a number for a place I had already been in contact with. That night, after discussing the day with my husband, we decided that attempting a diet could not hurt our child. As we purchased the expensive diet kit, which looked like it would increase our food bill by dramatic proportions, we said a prayer that this would be what we were finally looking for.

My husband and I decided that we would attempt to follow this diet for twelve weeks before making any other appointments, and we would follow it with no cheating. The first week our grocery bill tripled as I had to re-purchase all of our food staples. On this diet, Gracin was not allowed to eat any of his favorite fruits, and he was very upset. That was his biggest complaint: no berries. He loved strawberries and blueberries, and we had to replace them with pears.

As we sat there eating our first "new" meal, all I could think about was when Gracin was two months old and how he would stare at me whenever I was eating, following my fork with his eyes. It was as if I was eating gold, and he could not take his eyes off of it. I attempted to wait the six months as the doctored suggested, but, one day, when he was around three months old, he stole mashed potatoes off my plate, and that was the end of his waiting game. He made it known that he wanted food after that and would loudly object if you did not feed him food from the table. I believe he would have eaten until he exploded if we had let him. He cherished the time that he ate, and I would always worry that his tummy would get too full. My little baby turned into a very healthy plump child by his first year of age who devoured any type

Sensitivities, Frustration, and Finally Enlightenment

of food that you could imagine, especially fruit. I just did not understand how we got to where we were, eating bland food with no sugar, no white flour, and basically no sweetener at all.

After eating this diet for eight weeks, writing down symptoms, actions, and every detail of our day, we had had enough. We did not see any changes in our son's behavior other than him begging for his berries countless times a day. I felt distraught as I looked into all the recipes and came across the only allowed option for anything to appease our son: pizza. With not intending to put our family over the edge, I served the homemade pizza only to watch it be spit out shortly after the first bite. That was it. We had attempted the diet, and we felt as if we failed again. There was no improvement in Gracin's behavior. The food turned our stomachs. We were done. Although I do have to admit that even though most of the food was manageable, there just is nothing like comfort food.

In reality, I am not sure who objected more to the diet, but one thing was for sure, we could not keep eating like this. As I followed Gracin up the steps for bed that night, I noticed that he seemed more frail than usual. I walked my child into the bathroom and brought out the scale. My heart dropped as it showed that he had lost three pounds. I believe that book was thrown against the wall repeatedly after he went to bed as I once again felt let down. In an attempt to not blame the diet entirely, we had started to see that Gracin was becoming very particular to foods even before the diet began. At the time, though, we just chalked it up to his age and how most kids thin out around their third birthday.

With Gracin off to bed, my mind could not think about anything other than we needed help fast. Not only did he need help, but I also needed my child to eat again and gain back the weight that he lost. I also needed to talk to someone who could have an idea what was going on. We had now been on multiple specialist waiting lists for a total of four months. I felt there was no end in sight. The next morning I brought out the Pop Tarts that were hidden in the basement and let Gracin eat as much as his tummy could handle. We were completely done with any natural diets, but I did have some natural supplements that I had not tried. Not one of those worked at all in calming his symptoms, so I will not bore you with the details.

As time progressed, we still functioned in survival mode until, after almost five months, the phone rang. I finally received a call back from a pediatric specialist. Although I was elated about the call, I also felt very torn. As much as I wanted that appointment, I did not know what that appointment meant for our lives. It was Valentine's Day, and I decided a celebration was in order in an attempt to forget about all of our troubles. I made steak, mashed potatoes, green beans, and chocolate chip cookies for dessert. We had so much to celebrate as I announced, hidden in our cookies, that we were soon going to be a family of five. While Gracin smiled endlessly at knowing he would once again be a big brother, to our disbelief, he just stared at the food on his plate. He stated that the meat and green beans were too stringy, and the mashed potatoes were too mushy. We thought it was the diet that caused him to become a picky eater, but I believe the diet only masked him becoming sensitive to the textures in food.

At first we took a no nonsense approach where we basically stated that if you do not want to eat, then don't. Eventually he had to get hungry, right? Well we were shown how wrong we could be as we watched the weight drop off of him once again. We could no longer allow him to not eat, but we couldn't really force-feed a three year old either. Gradually, I accepted that there were just some foods that there was not any point in attempting to ask him to eat, such as mashed potatoes, green beans, warm cheese, and oranges. Really any food that had the "strings," as he called them, but as far as other foods that I knew did not "hurt" him as he stated, he was going to eat even if it meant that he had to sit there for a while.

He was going to eat some sort of a balanced diet because losing weight could not be an option for our growing child. Even though I said that I would never force my children to eat their food, a point is eventually reached where a parent must do what is best for their child's benefit. We had to make decisions to keep him healthy even if other people disagreed with our tactics. Ultimately, we had to block out all of the negative reactions from other people because we had to live with this child, and we knew him better than anyone else. Sadly, this decision was only one of many hard choices we had to choose to implement for our son's future gain.

As we prepared for yet another appointment, I tried to prep Gracin before we walked in the doors. I was no longer excited at the possibilities after we crashed and burned on the diet from the last doctor, yet I knew someone had to have the answers. My prepping was pointless as he became overwhelmed the second we stepped foot in the busy office. I was torn in so very many respects as I sat in yet another waiting room with my busy child who took full authority over his audience. I was expecting some sort of a decision on a diagnosis from this pediatric specialist, and my mind pondered what else my child could be diagnosed with other than ADHD.

Again, out in public I cannot even begin to express how awful of a parent I felt I appeared to be. My son either had to be held down or he would be, against my every instruction, climbing up on the laps of strangers or on tables, counters, and the like. Needless to say, by the time we were called, I was just so thankful to be in our own room. I did not care how long we had to wait in that tiny room. Although, Gracin had multiple ideas of how best to push me to my breaking point. I know he never intended to make me feel like I was losing control, but at the time, that is all it felt like: an attack on me.

As I sat in the examination room, with my chair in front of the door, Gracin ran around the room, climbing on the sink, trying to turn off the lights, and he even licked the floor countless times. Holding my youngest in my arms, feeling as though there was truly no point at attempting to stop Gracin, I rested my head on the door, closed my eyes, and felt the tears stream down my cheeks until the doctor knocked on the door. In the split second that followed the knock, Gracin's attention was averted as he ran to the door to greet the doctor with a one sided conversation about all the details of our waiting experience, his full name, address, phone number, my maiden name….until the doctor finally spoke.

Repositioning my chair again in front of the door, with my hand now also over the light switch, I fought for my turn to talk while Gracin simultaneously attempted with all of his might to turn out the lights. He did all of this while endlessly laughing. I explained the best I could about Gracin to the doctor. It was as if he were a racket ball sent flying throughout a room, except my child never ran out of momentum. I expressed that I felt anguish and embarrassment in not being able to control my son. However, I believe it was written all over my face and did not need to be verbally expressed.

Frankly, by the end of our half hour appointment, the doctor reluctantly expressed to me that my son had one of the worst cases of ADHD that he had ever seen. In an attempt to ease my mind, he assured me that it was not due to lack of discipline on my part. As this pediatrician continued to wipe the sweat from his forehead, he

Sensitivities, Frustration, and Finally Enlightenment

stated that he unfortunately was not able to give us any real answers at that moment. He knew Gracin had ADHD, but he was not willing to diagnose or prescribe medication to a child under five years of age. He stated that he wanted to call in a referral to one of the best psychiatrists in our county who dealt with children between the ages of three and five.

The doctor proceeded to try to convince me to take the appointment as he told me that he also thought there may be something else going on psychologically with our son. Sadly, his words felt basically the same as we had heard in the last appointment. He, personally, could do nothing to help us. In that moment, I needed no persuading. I had accepted that we needed help, and no convincing was in order. I was so incredibly thankful that we were finally going to get to the bottom of Gracin's behaviors even if it took yet another doctor to do just that. I felt such relief now that two different doctors, outside of our family, saw my son's activity level and agreed that this child was not the norm. I expressed my appreciation to the doctor as we finally opened the door that I was so diligently holding closed.

The reality was extremely hard to swallow, yet after feeling like I was the problem for so long, I was optimistic for the next appointment. I did not need to accept that this was just how kids were. I knew kids were not meant to be this hard, and I was elated that a professional finally saw it too. I had no real idea what a diagnosis meant, so, at the time, I do not know what I really expected to gain by getting one, but the process itself seemed to ease my mind. Thankfully, the pediatrician we had just met with must had pulled some major strings because we had our next appointment within a month's time.

As we waited, winter's final transition into spring warmed our spirits. We felt so optimistic if not for any other reason than being able to go outside again. I was thankful for the weather, but I had no idea what new behaviors were budding inside Gracin. Our son outright refused to step out of our back door because of what seemed like just about every reason that he could come up with. With just the change of the seasons, he had developed new fears of insects, most importantly bees. At the same time, he became convinced that he needed sunglasses all of the time because the sun "hurt" him. These behaviors were only some of the countless things that were now able to send his little body into screaming fits that were like unending tantrums. These lengthy episodes became a new norm as spring went into full bloom. Any small change at all did our little one in, and we knew all the more that we needed guidance.

At first, as these vast episodes escalated, we initially tried to stay with him to calm his rushing mind. However, we quickly realized that was the opposite of what he needed. Against everything in my upbringing, what felt correct in my deepest feelings and what I longed to do, I had to teach my son to calm down on his own. This was very hard for me because I wanted to wrap my arms around my child and let my loving embrace be enough. Gracin would punch, kick, bite, and scream endlessly until he, like a light switch, decided he was done. It was in that instant change that we realized it had to be up to him to stop. It was our loving control over our child that made us realize we had to help him develop the techniques in himself to calm his body during what was later coined a "meltdown." We felt we had such an angry little boy on our hands, and we had no idea what to do with him other than to walk away.

Of course, leaving him alone was not an easy to come by decision. One of the first things we did was stay with him during his screaming fit while giving him love and support. His anger

Sensitivities, Frustration, and Finally Enlightenment

only escalated with our presence. In addition, not only did the screaming at the top of his lungs eventually get to us after a period of time, but I also felt myself start to feel angry. That anger was directed at myself as well as towards Gracin after being in a room for a significant period of time hearing screaming and dodging kicks, punches, and bites. We were getting nowhere simply sitting in a room with him, and after a few weeks of feeling the anger build up inside, we had to shut the door and leave him to himself. I felt awful leaving him to his own devices, yet his anger was so intense that when he was immersed in his meltdown state, there was no calming him down. There was only experiencing with him.

Since showing our love was clearly not enough in this circumstance, we tried carrying him to a safe room where he could not hurt himself or anyone else around him. We would explain to him sternly and with no expression that we loved him so as not to increase his overwhelmed feeling. We would state that he had to stay in this room until he was ready to calm down and come out. Gracin was then left alone only with his security blanket, which he called "Puppy," and we would sit outside the door holding it shut. This worked at first, until he started kicking and punching holes in the walls while screaming even more at the top of his lungs. His puppy was clearly not enough to calm him down. It was a pathetic sight to see, from both sides of the door. I found myself sitting outside the door, holding it shut while crying and cradling my infant baby on my lap, while the child on the other side of the door was banging, kicking, and punching the wall, mattress, and himself over and over. I felt like a horrible parent. My eldest child was locked by himself in a room destroying everything that he could reach. One baby and one unborn baby were also ultimately hearing and feeling the stress of him melting down multiple times per a week.

We were reaching almost a daily over-stimulation pattern leading up to these meltdowns when, out of exhaustion and sleep desperation, my husband left a rosary in the room we called his calm-down room. Since he was experiencing, feeling, and expressing the only way his little body knew how to, I was left to figure out how to retrain his brain to experience something other than aggression. To no credit of my own, God led us to the answer. As I began to again prepare myself to sit outside his door, trying my best to not yell back at him, Gracin slowly stopped himself from his next screaming fit within only ten minutes time. Gracin proceeded in his over stimulated state to scream, then say a few calm words that we could not make out, and then continue the pattern. At first we had no idea what he was doing in the middle of screaming, but while watching him on the monitor, we realized he was calming himself down with prayer.

Within twenty minutes, he knocked on the door informing me he was done. When he walked out of the room holding his puppy and a rosary, I stood in disbelief. During the next few days, he would scream and cry for ten or so minutes, and then he would pick up his rosary and begin to recite the prayers. We would then begin to hear him calm down slowly as he caught his breath amidst the prayers. It was, in fact, our little miracle. Although we could not show him love in the ways we felt he needed, we were led by our prayer to teach him a way to calm himself on his own. We were not only experiencing much calmer days, but we were experiencing healing in all of our lives. Such a small repetitious act was calming our son once again, just as it had done for his sleep. I no longer had to hold the door shut during his meltdowns, which never lasted longer than twenty minutes at the point of escalation. It felt so nice to finally feel like we had done something right.

Sensitivities, Frustration, and Finally Enlightenment

Thankfully, we were not left to our own devices for much longer as the day finally approached for our appointment with the psychiatrist, and I felt a whole mix of emotions. My body shook as I pulled into the parking lot, said a silent prayer, and mustered the courage to begin the next step on our journey. Walking through the sliding double doors, I was presented with a pile of forms to complete. I stood at the reception desk trying my best to focus on which forms I needed to do what with. All the while, Gracin was attempting to climb up my leg, simultaneously pulling off my pants on purpose.

Sitting down to fill out countless papers, I felt helpless to control him from opening every door, standing on the chairs, crawling under the chairs, running around laughing to himself, exploring the waiting room bathroom, pushing the elevator button, or anything else that he deemed necessary. As I sighed helplessly, I made the executive decision to block out his actions. I could have attempted to stop him from moving constantly, but what was really the point, especially in that office. I had no desire to once again appear as the crazy mother who could not control her own child. In my own mind, those receptionists must have already seen everything, so who was I to worry what they thought of us? Whether I appeared as the crazy mother who chased, corrected, and looked frustrated, or the neglectful, aloof, inobservant mother who sat and played with her other child, I did not care. Facts as they were, we were sitting in a psychiatrist's waiting room, and no matter how you observed us, we appeared as quite an interesting sight to see. Either way, I thought I was going crazy from the over stimulation, but at least, in this moment, we were finally in the one place I felt secure in seeking help.

After the paperwork was completed, I sat in the waiting room contemplating what could be said this time. Based on what the last two doctors had said, I felt we may be getting an ADHD diagnosis again, but I really had no idea. I did not care completely what was going to be said to me. I only prayed that it would a short time until I could sit on the floor and play with my young son. I craved to enjoy his presence instead of being overwhelmed by it, which was ultimately why we were on this journey in the first place.

When we were finally called, Gracin shot like a cannon to the elevator door. He was elated with joy to finally be allowed to press the glorious button that he had been eyeing up from the moment we entered the waiting room. He pressed the button repeatedly until the door gradually opened at a snail's pace. Since Gracin did not let anything happen slowly, he helped the door open with all of his strength, and then he dashed inside. Standing in the elevator, the last year flashed before my eyes. As the elevator ascended to the next floor, my mind was in another place while my one hand firmly grasped my little man's arm. It felt like we had been on this journey for so long, and the last six months had been an eternity waiting for answers.

Our new psychiatrist greeted us as we stepped off of the elevator. Gracin ran ahead of us, breaking free of my grip and into the opened door at the end of the hallway. Her presence did not change as she just observed my child and, as a result, left me feeling calm and in a state of wonder at what she was thinking about my son. As she led me into her room, her eyes never left Gracin. I cannot express how, for the first time in my life, I was feeling relief in his behaviors, not because of what he was doing, but that she was seeing him for who he truly was. Even though he was standing on her couch, crawling under her desk, touching and moving every object in her room to his liking, and asking no telling - her ten million questions, I just sat there watching and waiting for her to finally say something. I took a deep breath as she

Sensitivities, Frustration, and Finally Enlightenment

began to speak to me for the first time. I was overwhelmed immediately by what she had to say when I heard not one but three diagnoses; two of which hurt to my very core.

The first that she explained to me was Asperger's. The *DSM-5*, which defines all mental disorders, now categorizes Asperger's as an Autism Spectrum Disorder, which renamed Asperger's to High Functioning Autism. This neurological diagnosis was extremely difficult to take. After being fully explained to me, though, I chose to accept it.

The second term she explained to me was a behavioral diagnosis and something that was rarely used in young children such as Gracin; although she felt this diagnosis described Gracin's meltdowns and impulsive thoughts quite well. That term is Intermittent Explosive Disorder or IED. I was a very confused before it was explained fully, but that also made sense given his behaviors.

Lastly, as we had expected, the ADHD or Attention Deficit Hyperactivity Disorder was stated, and it was explained as being a neurological diagnosis. This was of no surprise since it was not a term being presented to me for the first time, and I had already accepted it in my mind. The next thing I knew, I was being handed three different prescriptions to give to my little three year old child. Two were for his ADHD, and one was a sleep aid. As I stared at the prescriptions in hand, doubting if I wanted to give my son these pills, I graciously thanked the doctor for her time and expertise, and we said our goodbyes until the next appointment in only a week's time.

Walking down the hallway and into the elevator, I had a whole swarm of emotions begin to overwhelm by body. I felt nauseous, very warm, and my head pounded. Looking down at my firstborn son, I bent over to ask him for the hug I so desperately needed, to which he responded, "No thank you, Mommy!" I felt so distraught as I stood there with my arms outstretched for my child, yet I was left with my heart feeling stomped upon.

My happy, but temperamental, little fireball did not intend to leave me feeling this way. I concretely knew now that Gracin had something wired differently in his brain. He was not a brat or a child who was undisciplined. He was an atypical child, or a child who could be categorized as special needs. Gracin was not a typically developing child, and as I wrapped my head around the thought that he really never was as every other child appeared to be in my mind, his entire life finally made sense. Of course, I always felt different from every other parent I had talked to. I wasn't raising a child like all of my acquaintances were; I was raising a special needs child.

Still, though, I wanted love to be enough, and I was hurt that a simple hug was not something he mutually desired! Transferring my deep need for a hug into the infant in my arms, I felt like all the walls were collapsing around us while simultaneously opening up to a whole new realm for our future. As the elevator consequently interrupted the mountain of thoughts piling into my head, with the doors spreading open, Gracin galloped out the door, through the waiting room, the automatic sliding doors, and into the parking lot. Catching him literally seconds from a possibly huge disaster, I again was reminded that this child needed me now more than ever. All of my emotions were difficult to interpret, and, even though we got the diagnoses we desired, we received a whole lot more. My heart was heavy as I held back the tears until we were safely buckled into the car, where I cried.

Sitting in the parking lot with Mozart on for the kids, I called my husband at work. I could barely breathe. After a few minutes, I was able to contain myself enough to tell him what we were

Sensitivities, Frustration, and Finally Enlightenment

dealing with. Even though we were relieved at finally knowing, we felt such sadness for our son's future. We loved him so deeply, and we wanted so much more for him than daily pills and lifelong therapy.

My internal balance was off as I hung up the phone, started the car, and put it in reverse. I was in a mental spiral of grief until I glanced into the rear view mirror to witness my two sons laughing and smiling at each other. In that moment, I was immediately thankful that Gracin had a sibling. Not only did he have my husband and me behind him, but he was also going to have siblings to care for him through a lifelong bond that would extend far beyond my life's end. I was again reminded of the beauty in this life. I was not required to have all of this figured out. It was already in God's hands, and that is where I just had to leave it. I would soon have three wonderfully perfect children, and regardless of what diagnosis all of them potentially held, it was my job to pull myself together and be strong in order to best help my children.

I vowed at that moment to do exactly that, and over the next few weeks, our lives drastically changed again. We were informed that Gracin qualified to receive weekly therapy sessions in our home in addition to his new medications. On top of that, we had lots to talk about and consider for our future family. We had to not only inform our families of Gracin's neurological and behavioral diagnoses but also that our family was expanding again. On top of that mountain of information, we still had no idea what we should do with the medication that occupied our kitchen cabinet. Yet, as the days passed, we concluded that we knew he had to take them for his and our wellbeing.

We were overwhelmed with the information that was being tossed at us, yet my mind would not let me stop reading the pile of books I had purchased regarding Gracin's diagnoses. The most informative book that I found on the topic was *The Complete Guide to Asperger's Syndrome* by Tony Attwood. Within its pages, my son's entire life, as well as many aspects of my own life, seemed to be shared in almost every chapter.

I was captivated with the inventor, if you will, of the whole condition. The man's name was Hans Asperger, and he was quoted in 1944 as saying, "One can spot such children instantly. They are recognizable from small details, for instance, the way they enter the consulting room at their first visit, their behavior in the first few moments and the first words they utter." I found the whole diagnostic criteria fascinating as I, in fact, saw numerous traits present in one entire side of my family. I was amazed to read in Attwood's book that, "Recent research has indicated that 46 per cent of the first-degree relatives of a child with Asperger's syndrome have a similar profile of abilities and behaviors of a child with Asperger's syndrome, although usually to a degree that is sub-clinical, i.e. more a description of personality than a syndrome or disorder." I just could not stop reading. I was amazed that Hans Asperger also found a connection with attention problems. As stated in Attwood's book, "...at least 75 per cent of children with Asperger's syndrome also have a profile of learning abilities indicative of an additional diagnosis of Attention Deficit Disorder."

Gracin fit the Autism Spectrum Disorder, which included low functioning as well as high functioning children, perfectly under a large spectrum of a certain neurological criteria. Although I had felt alone in my thoughts and struggles for so long, I now felt as if we finally fit in somewhere. I certainly had a lot to learn, but I saw that the feelings of our extended families were very different. Our families had an especially hard time acknowledging the special needs diagnoses that made us feel accepted.

Sensitivities, Frustration, and Finally Enlightenment

Even though I found a bit of relief in knowing we could finally get help for our little lightning bolt, a whole new dimension quickly began to unravel. All the plans that a parent creates in their mind during the growth of their unborn child came to a screeching halt as a new reality began to emerge. With the diagnoses, I was led to finally discover why I always felt as if my typical parenting strategies were failing my own child in the physical world. Everything began to make sense: why my infant could not sleep soundly, why the wind made him scream, why he had such a fascination with strange objects, and countless other scenarios.

We were clearly not an anomaly; there were a lot of other families battling in what felt like a climb into the unknown. One of the hardest obstacles I found in raising Gracin was learning how to navigate the perceptions of others. Another obstacle was dealing with the media's portrayal of a perfect life. I needed to accept that I could not focus on a fairytale life of having sweet children who grow up with all smiles and giggles. It felt like a constant bombardment into our faces of the life we would never have.

I had come to realize I now needed to change my thought process in order to adapt for the child that I had been given. The vision that I always imagined was now, in effect, a farfetched reality, and that reason alone can leave a parent in total heartbreak for the shock it inevitably bestows upon a family. Slowly the shock does wear off as a caregiver nevertheless learns to shake the selfish feelings of what is happening to themselves and transfers that energy onto helping their special needs child. As we constructively transferred our negative energy into a positive one, we decided to figure out a way to explain the information to our families. We wanted a concrete way to describe everything we had learned in the last six months without forgetting anything and providing a future reference. The only way we knew how to do that was in written form.

I started by writing out an informative letter to present to the people within and closest to our family. This letter explained what we had recently discovered about Gracin. We read it to them word by word as most of them sat silently looking at us as if they either wanted to cry, cut us off to argue, or walk away. No one wanted to hear what we had to tell them, but the facts were as they were. We did not want to be doing this, but with Gracin's best interest in mind, we had to be strong. (See Appendix C: Family Explanation Letter).

This was not as well received from various individuals as I had hoped, but, with time, the diagnoses became easier to grasp, and I felt that our letter was the best way to explain everything. We understood that as a family to such a young child, it can be extremely painful for a person to embrace a diagnosis such as Autism, but it was because of that "label," if you will, that we were able to provide the best care for him. All children are different, and each child needs their own plan while embracing differences. Autism is, in reality, just a different type of brain wiring and ultimately just a different type of child.

It was our job as parents to make the best decision that we could for our son and for our immediate family's wellbeing and that reason alone was why we eventually chose the medication route. In my mind, I had tried the diets, the natural medications, allergy testing, and in the end, we saw no improvement. (See Appendix D: 1st Week of Medication).

Thankfully we saw a vast improvement in Gracin's behavior by only the third day on the medication. Our little boy was able to be a little boy and play. Although it was an extremely difficult decision to put my young son on medication, I can fully state that

Sensitivities, Frustration, and Finally Enlightenment

the medication was a much needed aid to saving our family dynamic. It brought us peace. It still brings tears to my eyes as I reread my own notes because my son's brain was finally able to be calmed enough to do what most child are blessed at being able to do from early on: play.

Most parents take play for granted, but I can guarantee you one thing: I never do. I thank God every moment that I catch my son playing with a toy, even if is a total mess, because during Gracin's first three years of life, I feel his play was stolen from him. I believe every parent deserves to watch their child immersed in play; it is truly a wonderful activity. I cannot fully express the joy that I experienced in my children's eyes as they were playing together enjoying each other's company for truly the first time enthralled in what children are meant to do best. In the words of Maria Montessori, "Play is the work of the child," and I was thrilled to witness my oldest child finally "working" like a child.

Chapter 16:
Not for the Weak of Heart

Child rearing, in my opinion, is not for the weak of heart. Raising a child, truly sacrificing for that child, I believe, changes a parent more than they ever expected. This reason, in itself, is why I feel that every parent needs to read real life accounts of how others worked through all of the stages of development and also how ultimate sacrifice on a child's behalf is the greatest gift. I honestly cannot explain where in my life I found the time to read during the months that followed the diagnosis of my Gracin, but I was determined to soak up as much knowledge on his diagnoses, as well as what it meant to love genuinely, that I could find.

St Catherine of Siena, one of only three women in the Roman Catholic Church given the formal title of Doctor of the Church, while in a dialogue with God learned that, "The willing desire to suffer every pain and hardship even to the point of death for the salvation of souls is very pleasing to me. The more you bear, the more you show your love for me." I was astounded at what I read and how I interpreted these very "heavy" conversations that she was gifted to have. I hoped my suffering and my day to day in and out trials with my special needs child could perfect not only my soul but also that my good works could be offered up for other souls as well. I felt as if I was given a gift, an intense one but nevertheless a gift, that my life could help others through my own trials and sufferings in raising this unique child. I was no longer saddened by the outlook of my life; I was invigorated. As hard a message as it was to accept and understand, within the pages I continued to read, "The soul, therefore who chooses to love me must also choose to suffer for me anything at all that I give her. Patience is not proved except in suffering, and patience is one with charity, as has been said. Endure courageously, then." The message was clear in my mind. In St. Catherine of Siena's dialogue with Christ in her ecstasy, which provided her with a one-on-one conversation with God, himself, I had heard exactly what I needed in regards to patience, courage, and charity. Therefore, I felt I was given a way into finding how to suffer in this world in order to gain in the virtues that I had always lacked and needed for my own spiritual growth. All of the prayers of my life were ultimately being answered after all, just not in the way I desired them to be answered but in God's will for my life.

Within the same month, I stumbled across a blog on the internet entitled, "Why I Should Have Never Had Eight Children." This title is a little deceiving, that the author should really not have had her children. It is really about what those children were meant by coming into existence: "The souls in your life are gifts, each of whom is meant to sanctify you in a particular way. My little sanctifiers are the artisans who change and mold me in all the ways God knows I need, and they are their father's and their siblings' artisans, too." Therefore, how selfish was I being in believing that God was not hearing my prayers? Though, as I sat in my bedroom during night's quietest of hours, I was led to understand from multiple sources that as the parents of a special needs child, my husband and I were being given a unique opportunity to grow spiritually.

This job is not for the weak, but regardless of how strong I ever believed myself to be, it was now time for me to develop my ultimate capacity for growth in love. When you really think about it, it is amazing how many ways there are of dealing with the same childhood issues in the various ways of parenting. The most important way that I learned for parenting was giving my one hundred percent devotion to the tiny little human who grew in my womb before I ever even knew he was there.

Parents must constantly tweak their parenting style to choose the methods that work best for their own child and family each given day. If those styles are based on a selfless devotion to the child, a parent will never fail. In a gene study conducted in November of 2014 entitled, "A Fresh Take on Autism's Diversity," geneticist David Ledbetter, chief scientific officer at Geisinger Health System in Danville, Pennsylvania states that, "What we've learned in the last five years about the underlying genetics is that there are hundreds, if not a thousand or more, different genetic subtypes of autism."

It seems daunting based on the above mentioned information to then state that there is one best way to guide a child diagnosed with a broad term such as autism. My son's autism could be just one of thousands of different types that are caused by some sort of genetic mutation in the coding that intertwined at his conception. In the same article, it also mentions that, "microarray technology revealed that people with autism tend to carry many copy number variations, deletions or duplications of large stretches of DNA that encompass multiple genes. Researchers soon saw that people who harbor the same copy number variants often share other characteristics and symptoms as well." It is then a relieving thought to hear, once again, that my son is not the way he is because I did something wrong during my pregnancy or within the first few years of his upbringing. It is conclusively just one of the things that happened in the coding of his genetic makeup that caused my son's brain to be developed differently. Again, this was never something I did to my son, as I and many others have thought, that we, as parents of a child with autism, did something to have our children become this way.

Many times I struggled with how to discipline my child because I did not know what was at the root of his behavior pattern. The question constantly was in my mind if each behavior was typical or if it was something that he could not control because of how his brain was specifically made. Some issues I needed to take more care in approaching compared to others, and that confused some family members. Sleep was one of those examples. It became a major disagreement for the vast majority of our family members who did not understand why we did things the way we chose to do them. I was constantly told on all fronts, that children will sleep when they are tired. It is a good thing that I just could not accept that. I knew my own unique child, and the way in which his brain worked would never had allowed him to sleep deeply if I had permitted him to make his own bedtime decisions. Gracin craved structure and routine, and it was my job to provide him with the correct atmosphere even if I had to disagree with everyone around me. I felt the element of a schedule brought us all peace and was of the utmost importance in our lives.

As the months unfolded, we were met head on with our son's intermittent explosive behavior, and I constantly thanked God that we established Gracin on a routine when we did at just over a year of age. We officially renamed his tantrums into meltdowns, and they were the most challenging and frustrating part of his progression. Finally, by the end of Gracin's 3rd year, we had our schedule mastered, and Gracin always knew what would happen next. He felt security in his life even though we were faced with the impossible challenge of explaining to a three year old that sometimes life gives us things we cannot prepare for. In those moments, our house would come to a screeching halt as life no longer appeared calm.

We received a lot of stares and criticism from many different sources during and after a meltdown. I, myself, was becoming over stimulated from the amount of energy and time I was providing into controlling my son's environment. Consequently, a few doctors suggested I start an anxiety medication. I felt the risks were too high for my growing family, so I kindly declined, but I will never fault anyone who believes they are dealing with too much. At times, life seemed all too much to bear. We had the minutes scheduled, and we followed the clock to almost a fault, and, yes, it was incredibly hard, but oh so needed. I felt so much tension that at times I felt I could not enjoy my children or the world around me. That is one of my main regrets of Gracin's year of being three. With the constant reminder of what life is ultimately meant to be - a continual perfecting of our souls for our ultimate destination - I was comforted. I used myself as a tool to do everything in my power to establish an environment that was calming for Gracin. I took total control over our schedule, limited our visitors, and made sure that he felt loved in the ways that his body needed. In essence, I let him be in total control so that, in time, we could help him learn to accept changes in his routine without a meltdown. Escalation and control seemed as if they were Gracin's favorite things to do; although, it was the only thing I believed he was actually able of communicating in the moments of overstimulation.

With time, struggle, prayer, repetitiously identical days, and perseverance the child who emerged from his shell is an amazing sight to see. Our love had to be changed in order for our Gracin to excel, but because no one's capacity for love is the same, it was not an unreasonable expectation. These special needs children are special not because their diagnosis deems them as inferior and their brains or their bodies are developed differently. They are special because they are God's way of perfecting our world's love within their lives. I believe they are a beautiful sight in the grand scheme of things, not only because they truly teach us what it means to love, but also because they will be some of the first souls to welcome us at the heavenly gates. I genuinely believe that the special needs individuals of this world are God's little caterpillars who, although seem to be stuck in a cocoon in their lives here on earth, will emerge in the next life as the most beautiful souls upon whom we have ever laid eyes.

Part 5:
Surrendering

Chapter 17:
In Sight of the Summit

Grasping the wet and glassy cliffside, I became invigorated by the sunlight. It felt refreshing and revitalizing to definitively see the visible rock mass above me. This allowed me to easily differentiate the next sturdiest rock of which to take hold. As I pushed my body forward and felt the rhythmic pitter-patter of raindrops, they became a calming agent, compared to previously appearing as a distraction.

Our bodies were noticeably worn down by the brutality of the hurricane that continued to hover over the beach. Although, a calm was beginning to become increasingly present upon the atmosphere. The wind had died down significantly into a swift but less than harmful blow, and it seemed conclusively as if we were finally experiencing the last of this passing storm. It even seemed that the grip of my child began to become sturdier as he discovered how to hold on differently, while seemingly accepting a sense of security with his mother's intentions.

I visualized climbing relatively effortlessly amongst the rocks ahead. However, as I became distracted in my own desires, my footing slipped for the first time. Watching a small rock break free and plummet down into the ocean below, bypassing my lifeguard by only a fraction of space, I gasped at the sight below me.

Freezing unintentionally in my place upon this gigantic rock, my mind spun out of control with dismal thoughts.

Attempting my best to pay no attention to my own bodily ailments by overpowering my mind, we continued on our climb. However, I felt as if my frame was collapsing with each change in position. It seemed as if the small breaks, which we had found upon our journey, were not quite long enough. I moved onward at a snail's pace until I felt a warm nudge on my shoulder as our lifeguard informed me of another spot to rest our worn down bodies. Assembling all of my courage, I followed behind him rapidly as we were led to safety in a cave nestled in the high shelf upon what felt like our prison. Resting my body alongside my son's, we relaxed in the dark and hidden seclusion of our shelter before we had to once more resume our upward ascent.

Watching the rain fall and the ocean roar in the distance, I coaxed my child to rest his eyes as I rocked his body into a deep sleep. As he slept, I saw him relax totally and dream as I invoked multiple prayers of thanks to my creator. With an array of peace sweeping throughout the surrounding darkened restoration, our bodies were able to recover as they desired. Allowing my mind to fall into a restorative nap, I dreamt of a life, ironically not much different than the one I currently possessed.

Regrettably awakening before my dream had fully concluded, I was now even more determined to finish our climb. I looked upward from out of our shelter only to be blinded by the sun that had reached its apex in the sky. Surrendering all trust into God's hands once again, we cautiously began to blindly advance on our journey. To my astonishment, the rain had changed into a light misty drizzle, and for the first time in what felt like a lifetime, my hair began to gradually dry in the warmth of the sun. Feeling as if I was no longer held back by my own fears of what lay ahead, I

In Sight of the Summit

readily pushed my body to its maximum capacity. With minimal breaks and only encountering a handful of additional ledges for rest, we pushed onward.

Reaching with my one free arm for what I thought would be my next hold, I felt an unfamiliar flat surface. My spirit was lifted in amazement. Praying to God that I contained the strength to elevate my own body weight as well as my son's onto the summit of the cliff, I gathered what courage I had left from the depths of my mind. I invoked one final push from the current rock that held my footing; I was in awe as I elevated us onto the top of the mountain. Lying on the soft bed of grass, I reached below to help our lifeguard to the peak of elevation as we collapsed backward into an array of laughter and tears that could not be contained.

♥

For most individuals there is always one specific season, which seems to feel as though it will never end; mine is winter. During my most depressing time of the year, the sun never seems to shine through the grey covered sky. Although I know it will end, it sometimes feels like it will go on forever. Life, in itself, seems to present a lot like the seasons, and because of this there will always be time periods in our lives that we must push through, no matter how much we do not want to, in order to get to the other side. In this respect, I feel this season analogy is the easiest scenario in order to relate what it is like to be the parent of a special needs child. Although impossible to fully comprehend what it exactly feels like raising a child with autism or a similar diagnosis, you can picture it somewhat if you just imagine your most difficult season of weather being extended indefinitely.

Thankfully, there is always a way to improve our lives. In our situation, the age of three was comparable to the worst cold and dark winter climb that we had ever known. However, we were on the path to improvement. Even though we had trial after trial with no warm air, birds, or flowers in sight, we believed we could transform our lives with perseverance. It may have seemed as if we were stuck on what felt like a cold and dark mountainous climb into the unknown, one that attempted to suck the happiness and the love of life right from us. We were truly not. In reality, along with our continuous prayers and actions, we were witnessing our lives transforming for the better with each step forward.

As time progressed, the sky eventually began to clear, the birds slowly returned, some color even popped up from the ground, and combined with some warm air gusts hurled our way, we were led to the top of our mountain. To be fair, I am not sure to whom I can even credit our child's immense changes. I certainly cannot and will not take all of the credit and say it was because of what we did as parents. I say this because we were only led to do what we were doing in our actions and perseverance because of how we believed God desired us to push through the struggles using our faith.

Finally, and in God's time - never our own - we were led to find the ways to evolve from the heartbreak and trauma the diagnosis bestowed upon all of our lives. We were led to understand that even though our bodies had been wounded in the process, our spirit was fully intact and truly better than it ever was before as we declared our mission in this life to help our little boy become the best he could possibly be. This led the age of four to still feel as if it was an uphill climb, but it was a much easier climb compared to what we had previously endured.

Within the struggles of our seemingly impossible lifestyle, we were given the tools and the understanding as to why our son actually acted in the ways that he did. This led to our fourth year journey where we were steered to learn how to love our son in the exact ways that he needed us to love him, while helping him to adapt to new situations at the same time. It was by these precise ways that we were able to endure his behaviors day in and day out. Thus, we gradually became able to guide him into becoming a less rigid individual. At the same time, we secured our own internal happiness and hope in the situation in which we were gifted.

Growth in any area of our lives is not comfortable. In order to move forward, though, we must consequently push the edges of that comfort zone gradually to establish an end product. Within our hope, our love, and our trust, the product that emerged - our son - was and still is an amazing sight to see. Gratefully, as we watched the dark moments pass and discovered the apex of our mountainous climb, we felt like we were on top of the world.

Chapter 18:
Ready, Set, Let's Argue

"Gracin, my child, please just stop talking... Breathe in between words... Sometimes we think things without saying them... When I say no, it does not mean you can keep asking. The answer is no... You may not do this or that"... or ANYTHING! Gosh, I just sounded awful to myself and everyone around me. I felt terrible. How could it be that everything my child did be done in the wrong way? Why did his brain process everything in what seemed as a backwards manner?

To answer everyone's constant questions as well as my own, yet again, it was because this child was not the stereotypical norm that everyone expected him to be. Gracin could not be categorized by his outward appearance. It was easy to forget or push aside that he was, in fact, dissimilar to most other children. He may not have been blind, deaf, or physically impaired, yet with a careful eye one could see that he was incapable of making the same connections that most other children were. His diagnosis was a fact easily missed if you were too busy to see it or frankly did not want to see. Although, watching him intently, one could not deny the adversities. We, as his parents, were incapable of ignoring the facts as they were, and as difficult as those facts remained, Gracin needed those extra warnings, scheduled activities, and time, which proved that Gracin was vastly different than other children in his same age group.

As an effect of appearing so typical, most children did not know how to relate to him. Within minutes of initiating an encounter to play, they would simply just walk away from him. Gracin, unaffected by the other child ending their play abruptly, returned happily to whatever he was doing beforehand. I, though, was endlessly puzzled as these situations increased. Was it because they could not understand him, or did other children believe he was different from them? The thing that really amazed me was how quickly these other young ones came to the conclusion that Gracin was different. It was as if he was so overly friendly that other children just knew something was tainted. Gracin was different, but was it so apparent that it was unacceptable to befriend him even if only for a few moments at the park? I can only describe it as if he intruded into their personal space and brought them into their own feelings of insecurity, so they shunned him as a result. However, I really will never know why those children walked away so quickly from my son.

It was incredibly difficult because he was, and still is, so alike other children that he is deemed as "normal" just in his appearance. He then has this extra something buried beneath the skin that just pushes him into the special needs realm that most others cannot fully understand. All kids tire their parents out, but onlookers to our situation may never grasp what I am describing unless they have their own child on the autism spectrum or with a similar diagnosis.

It was astonishing to me that other children could pick up on his subtle differences easier than most adults ever could. To another adult, he was an interesting and fascinating child to speak with about a topic of his choosing. Upon further review of more than just a lengthy one-sided conversation of informative information on one of Gracin's favorite topics, the judgments were brought to light. I eventually heard comments such as that he was rude, obnoxious, out of control, or just plain spoiled. I received an extraordinary amount of criticism and glares from individuals I did not even know and some that I had known for a lifetime. I felt so torn because I wanted to talk to others about my son, yet I learned time after time not to even bother to try to talk to anyone about him outside the family, or sadly even within the family.

Though it was while attempting to explain what sets my child apart from another child of his same age, that I most certainly heard the typically coined response, "Well my child does that too," with the exact same attitude numerous times. Over and over, I was forced to bite my tongue in order to avoid yet another argument that would leave me flustered and feeling defeated. Ultimately, it led me to once again feel as if everyone around me was siding against us. I could only think to relate that yes, their child most likely does talk a lot, argue, get bored with toys, run in the house, and talk about their favorite things at inappropriate times, but it is to the intensity that our child does these actions that, nevertheless, sets him apart.

The constant ongoing opinions about how we were doing almost everything wrong was just too overbearing. There was no more sense in constantly arguing with the individuals in our lives. Consequently, in a desperate attempt to not feel hurt anymore, we essentially pulled everything in. It was a tragic conclusion to what I felt was something that brought enlightenment and acceptance in my own life yet pulled me away from the individuals who were supposed to support me and my family.

Accordingly and without remorse, I gave all of my being to Gracin and my other children. The time that my children were sleeping, I spent with my husband. When he was busy, I learned to occupy myself with reading as I ultimately became the bookworm that I should have been in high school but never had the motivation to be. I wrote notes upon notes instead of conversing with the outside world. I literally had all of my conversations written on scrap paper. In the deepest portion of my heart, I nearly acquired the isolation that I believe my child felt in order to better understand him.

The thing I found impossible to relate to anyone with spoken words was that I did not desire my child to be different from everyone around him. I had received that criticism countless times. I did not want to label him with a diagnosis per se, but I did believe that by having a label of explanation to his life, he could have tremendous growth with himself versus not having that same label.

I did not want him to be an outcast socially, yet it was obvious he was not a social butterfly. I did not understand the world's desire to attempt to push my child to conform to a set of social desires that were, in reality, unneeded. Even though he truly desired to be every child's friend, it was very obvious that other children did not share his same interests. As much as those peers seemed to stimulate his curiosity in their play, Gracin just could not sustain the same untimed play as they could. Their play bored him with its duration, and as an observer, it seemed that he was fighting a war within his own mind as to what his brain and his body would allow him to do simultaneously.

Though within the adult world, Gracin excelled. He could literally argue about anything. He practiced his potion on me infinite times per hour. He could argue with anyone a fact as simple as getting him a drink of water or feeding the cat. I was at such a loss, and it seemed that if he was not arguing, he was most certainly talking loudly.

If he believed it was an inappropriate time for me to have a drink, go to the bathroom, or even change his brother's diaper, I received a response typical of, "No, you need to do…," in the most condescending tone you can imagine. It was mind numbing to constantly have a young child not only try to tell you what you could and could not do, but then to also do it in such a harsh tone.

It was almost as if every single thought that popped into his head was vocalized and vocalized in a very condescending tone. It appeared that Gracin needed to have an opinion on every topic and without a doubt had to have the final word. He could not understand or fathom why he did not know everything or why he was not privileged to know everything. Justly, we were at a complete loss as how to help our child transform his words into a more respectful tone and become less of a dictator.

In all the typical parenting books that I felt were of no use to our child, I finally stumbled upon something that we could adapt to disciplining our son. As I have stated before, typical parenting strategies do not work on a child with high functioning autism. I believe one of the reasons why this is the case is that the connections in their brain have trouble retrieving information at the proper time. So, when they call upon their thoughts to help them decide what to do next, they are not always led towards the correct outcome. This term is defined as Executive Function, which is basically reasoning and problem solving. This is the exact reason why time outs never really worked for Gracin. On the one hand, he was not capable of sitting quietly for four minutes at his current age. Secondly, he was not able to remotely access why he was even in time out in the first place. Punishments were useless. He needed to be concretely guided time after time to retrain his brain to automatically connect how he should speak or act in any given situation.

As outlined in *Parenting with Grace* by Gregory and Lisa Popcak, we started having Gracin restate his statements immediately in a respectful tone, while attempting to stay calm ourselves, after he said something out of line. According to the Popcaks, "When children say something in an obnoxious way, use the restating technique by asking them to rephrase their statement or ask them to repeat a more appropriate phrase that you suggest to them." This was something that seemed redundant, yet slowly over time (we still use it daily) worked. It is extremely hard and does seem as an endless endeavor for us all, but in light of attempting to not take the first statement's tone as disrespect and accepting that his first comment is most likely caused by lack of proper brain connections, we made significant strides. We also did a similar technique with behavioral issues. This is labeled "do overs" by the Popcaks. They recommend that, "When you are trying to change some behavior in your child, you must have him practice a more appropriate alternative every time you catch him doing the inappropriate thing. This is the only way your child will get enough practice to change."

I believe that by doing these two techniques, a parent is not only becoming a more attentive and less selfish individual by devoting a large portion of their time to their child, but they are also guiding their children into becoming a wonderfully respectful and loving individual. The key is that you cannot take the first statement or action personally and as an attack on yourself. You must rise above the behavior or comment to look beyond the initial reaction for the progress with the second try. Over time, and yes this could mean years, your children will reset those inappropriate connections and learn to be what you are yourself modeling as guided selflessness and respect. With these two strategies as our ultimate guide, I felt I could conquer anything thrown at me.

As the age of four began to unfold, our name crept to the top of the list for services to start in our home. As excited as I was for these services to start, I quickly felt overwhelmed by the presence of outsiders in our lives multiple times per week. Gracin would become worse, much worse, after these individuals initially got to our home and within the days following their departure. It felt like an intrusion into his life, even though they meant to give us help and new ideas. For a child whose parents were, themselves, devoted to giving him all of our energy and devotion in life, the services provided by various agencies were just more things for him to have to get used to.

As a result, I quickly dropped all of the services that were aimed at giving me ideas instead of hands-on helping him. The services that we kept were only a few of the ones recommended. The ones I felt that were the most helpful for our exact situation were those provided by an occupational therapist and the special needs teacher who worked one-on-one with Gracin. I wished I had learned of these services sooner because I later realized these services are available to very young children.

Special needs services are a very touchy subject. Although they are put into your life with the aim to help an individual family, some individuals will most definitely clash with what a family's goals may be. It is a very difficult world to navigate through, but one thing I learned was to never be afraid to state my own needs.

Personally, I also felt that I had a better experience with a team of individuals who were older and more experienced than me and not fresh out of school. The reason for these individuals being in my home was purely based on need and not a friendship as I saw the younger therapists occasionally attempt to incorporate. There were very few individuals who fit into our lives, but those that did were a God send, and I am extremely thankful.

Though the facts will always remain that these children are yours and NOT theirs to do what they want with. Just because it is a government run program does not mean you have to accept it as being the best thing for your child. In *Early Intervention & Autism*, it states that, "What is important is how often you interact with your child…, not the number of professionals who stream in and out of our house. They can help, but *you*, the child's parents, who interact with him 24/7, it is *you* who make the real difference for the child." I believe that God was guiding me into the proper ways of raising my own child, and these individuals were just an aid in helping to get us where we needed to be. Justly, they did not need to be in our lives. It was my choice to allow them to be a helping presence in my home. If you truly believe that you cannot do this on your own and are willing to accept the help, then these special needs services are the best course of action in my opinion. Although, if you feel that they are a hindrance to how you are trying to raise your children, then you are free to decline or reduce the duration of those services at any time. They may have their Masters degree and the education behind the science of a special needs child, but as any dedicated parent, you have your PhD in your own child.

Life, I will admit, was not even close to easy. I was in constant spoken and unspoken multiple battles with family members who thought their tactics were better for Gracin. This was on top of my own child's battle of wills, which he felt he knew best. Then there was my own selfish battle in my head where my body fought for what it wanted, and my mind fought for the utmost devotion to my child. Coupled with all of that, we were increasing Gracin's medication every few months, and it was immensely frustrating.

Ready, Set, Let's Argue

The days following the increase, Gracin would be the poster child for calm, cool, and collected. Although, slowly but surely as his high metabolism got used to the new dosage, his behaviors slowly came back. It was never his focus that we first noticed dwindling. It was always his hyperactivity where he could not sit in one place without constantly moving about.

His sleep was the same. We would have significant strides for weeks at a time where he slept relatively soundly only awakening to go to the bathroom or to, "Tell us a question" once per night. Then, within a matter of just a few sleeps - as we called them - it seemed we took three steps back. Countless nights we would hear the toilet flush as Gracin fell into the wall multiple times and/or yelled that he peed on the floor once again. As he finally proceeded back to his bed, he would then have an almost yelling conversation with puppy - which he swore to us was his quiet voice - for twenty minutes before his body would take over and shut down once again.

Holding it all together was an art, but there were times that the arguing brought me down almost to rock bottom. I had daydreams, which I am reluctant to admit, where I duct taped his mouth shut, tied him to his bed, and took a long uninterrupted nap. Thankfully, my conscience would not allow me to do these things, and lots of self-talk, prayer, and phone calls to my husband at work calmed my overwhelmed mind. Countless times I was quite close to bottom, but because of my devoted husband and a select few individuals who I allowed close to us, I thankfully never reached that point.

As time moved forward, we were led to what we feel was the root of all of the arguing. I believe that our child truly did not fully grasp why there were so many variables in how we asked him to act. He thought in black and white, and we just were not explaining things to him in that same manner. For instance, if we told him we were getting ready to go to bed, please go to the bathroom, in his mind he felt he did not have to go right that moment, even if he may have to go in ten minutes, so an argument would erupt.

Asking things of Gracin was a lot easier on all of us after we learned to write down exactly what we were asking him to do including the time frame in which we expected the job to be done. It was by this way that we allowed his brain to easily process, without any question, the task he was expected to do without an escalating argument. Since Gracin argued because he could not understand why and how we were asking things of him, when he felt they were unnecessary, writing things out was our go to plan. It was now in his black and white, right or wrong mind frame. We had to be the ones to evolve our behaviors to again suit his needs.

Gracin did not argue because he did not want to do the tasks we were asking of him. I have come to believe it was because he honestly was not capable of having any trust in us whatsoever as other children do in their parents. His trust had to be proven and changed to what he could understand before he could readily follow through with a request from another person. Although I cannot state that he now trusts in our decisions entirely and does not argue all facts, I do feel at least we have found some ways to prove to him why he should ultimately trust us, even if it takes an undetermined period of time for that trust to be given.

In addition to these facts, if someone came over to our house either expected or unexpected, it seemed as if Gracin would immediately try to manipulate the environment and cause as many disruptions as he possibly could to prevent anyone from having a meaningful conversation. Upon further discovery, I realized that this was not what was going on at all. In *Ten Things Every Child with Autism Wishes You Knew*, Ellen Notbohm describes how a child attempts to establish control within their own environment by their behaviors:

> When so little is within their control, many children on the autism spectrum experience life as a continuous battle to hold onto whatever power they do have to direct their lives. Their attempts to control may be overt (confrontational, aggressive behavior that looks like defiance), or they may be passive-aggressive (they silently or covertly continue to do what they wish regardless of attempts at redirecting behavior). Your daily life as a typical adult flows in a perpetual, minute-by-minute stream of choices. You take for granted both the array of choices you have and your ability to act upon them. Such reasoning and decision-making skills are much more limited in your child with autism. What appears to be controlling behavior on your child's part can also be seen as evidence of her ability to think independently and affirm her own wants and needs. Channel these qualities as you work with her to instill decision-making skill and increase the number of choices and opportunities for success in her world.

This was one of the hardest and most embarrassing qualities in my son's young life. Once I accepted that he was not trying to make my life harder but just trying to regain control over the current unknown situation, we were led to vast understanding and, therefore, growth on both of our parts.

During these moments of unknown, it felt as if I had two choices to make in order to react to my child. I could give in and let the behavior happen; therefore acknowledging that he could get away with whatever he wanted. Or I could interrupt talking with our guest and control my child repeatedly. With either option, I felt as if I was letting someone down, but in choosing the latter, I was helping Gracin feel secure and not neglected. Even though I, myself, appeared as if I had to control everything about my child's life, in reality I had to help my son feel secure. If the person I was talking to could not understand the devotion I had to my child, then they did not belong in my home to begin with.

My goal was for the long term, and if the word discipline is ultimately defined as meaning to teach, then who was I to ignore each prime teaching moment. I only wish I had known of sensory integration therapy when my son was younger, so I could have helped him learn to calm his own bodily needs better than I was at that current time (See Appendix E: Sensory Integration Therapy). We, as parents, are obligated to give our children all of our being in order for them to succeed. This means not just being there where we have time and nothing else to do. I feel that we must sometimes deny our own needs in order to instruct our child, especially our special needs child.

Chapter 19:
The Life I Discovered is Ever Changing

Life never stays the same. Honestly, the only thing that you can guarantee in this life is that IT WILL change. This was something that almost everyone in my family would try to explain to me, in different variations, when as a little girl and I made vast plans for the future. Nevertheless, I blindly continued to plan for five, ten, and fifteen year increments amusingly expecting them to all fall together perfectly. Time and time again my plans fell out through the bottom, and I was left questioning what I could have possibly done wrong. Remembering back to those numerous conversations, I realize that I never heeded any of that advice until I had a child of my own.

As the years unfolded, my husband and I attempted to have control over the world within the walls of our home and our parenting regiment, yet I am not sure if we ever truly did. With each passing day, we were thrown new and different curve balls to which we had to adapt. Life, in itself, seemed to be out to get us on most days, and initially we felt that we were getting nowhere in helping our child. However, from an outsider's perspective, it was only because we did not see the big picture.

Over time, we evolved as we began to stop wishing that Gracin was different or thinking of what he could have been like if we would have done this or that differently. We began to cherish him just as he was. We found ways to rejoice in the tiny improvements that we were able to help him overcome, and, as a result, in the fourth year of his life, our lives began to seem less of a challenge.

Therefore, I learned to begin making goals for our future instead of plans, and seemingly those goals were more easily moved if they needed to be. We, as parents, were learning how to keep Gracin feeling safe, while at the same time accepting that we must also change in order to be what our child needed us to be. Consequently, Gracin began to feel more secure in the little bubble of a world that we created for him as he saw the devotion and the respect that we gave his individualized needs over time. This actualized process momentarily bestowed the calm into our lives that we had been searching for.

We began to prepare ourselves to slowly begin incorporating changes into Gracin's daily routine in order to help him break out of his shell. Although we honestly were so happy in all the progress that we had found, I will confess that we were not ready for another upheaval. Even so, despite our newfound niche of security, life had other ideas in mind as my water broke and we welcomed our third son into our lives.

As much as we desired our home to continue to be Gracin's calm, controlled, and safe place, our newborn had his own plans. We had hoped that our new baby would be another calm and laid back child, as was our second child, though that just was not in the cards. He was his own person and instantly made his own needs loudly known. As much as Gracin was enthralled in the excitement of having another sibling, which we prepared him for months in advance, this was, nevertheless, an upheaval into his environment. This was the first major disruption to our finally concretely predictable world, and it seemed to send us all running for cover.

The Life I Discovered is Ever Changing

The first few nights with our colicky newborn were by far the worst as this turmoil into Gracin's universe was enough to end every well-adjusted habit, including his sleep, which he possessed. Gracin's mind would not allow him to stay away from his new brother at any time period throughout the day but especially in the middle of the night. Even though for our new son's breathing benefit, most nights I slept in a rocking chair on the other side of the house, Gracin still made it a point to seek us out, hourly. Everything in his universe was upside down. We had a new person living with us, Mommy no longer slept in her bed, and if his new brother's eyes were open, he was crying.

Gracin found it necessary to investigate and inform us if his new brother was crying, if he had just stopped crying, or if he believed he needed a diaper change at 4:00 in the morning. It seemed that as soon as I finally got the baby back to sleep, or I finally fell asleep, Gracin came barging into the room just to tell me something that really did not need to be said. It was a mind-numbing process, and although we were happy for this new life, my husband and I felt as if we were being pushed to our ultimate breaking point of sleep deprivation and sanity. I felt as though this new change had ruined Gracin's security, yet after the first few months, our lives transformed immensely.

Gracin loved his baby brother with all of his being and desired to help calm him in every way he could, without my prompting. Gracin read piles of books to him while the baby was both asleep and awake, brought him anything that he thought the baby needed, and sang to him almost constantly to calm his endless cries. As much as Gracin's help was, in reality, not helpful, it was in those moments that he was learning how to think of another person other than himself. The birth of his brother had actually, without our knowledge, started teaching Gracin how to become selfless. I believe that it was because of this new life and the change that happened by his birth that Gracin slowly began to be molded into a more accepting individual.

Through the process of having an extremely needy baby brother, Gracin learned to quiet his actions down a small notch in order to help his new sibling sleep peacefully. Before our new addition, all it would take was one small change in Gracin's routine to send his body over the edge. Since the birth of our third child, he seemed to understand how important it was to give of himself for his brother's benefit. It was amazing to see this highly sensitive child attempt to console a baby who had his own set of extra needs, allowing Gracin to feel more helpful.

Although we saw amazing changes in how Gracin was accepting his new brother as a constant in our life, this was not what we felt would help him learn to accept abrupt split second variations with ease. We recognized that we had to take the first step in this process because we knew the kinds of meltdowns we were potentially in for. With starting an adjustment in schedule, we were skeptical as to when and how to best begin to incorporate these changes. I believe we were able to incorporate slow changes for our son while still helping him stay in some sort of control by the following ways.

As I have related previously, our typical day functioned in a strict format, and we hardly ever diverted from the plan. Here is what our day looked like on a Monday through Friday format:

7 a.m. - Awake and getting dressed for the day followed by a thirty minute show IF he followed all his sleep rules, within reason, all night long

8 a.m. - Breakfast followed by his medication

9 a.m. - Structured playtime along with constant monitoring - we tried to be outside as much as we could

The Life I Discovered is Ever Changing

10 a.m. - Organized learning including math, reading, and writing while listening to various composers

11 a.m. - Lunch

11:30 a.m. - Clean up time

Noon - Rest time

3 p.m. - Wake up time followed immediately by snack and a half an hour show if he followed his sleep rules during his nap

4 p.m. - Free playtime, typically outside

5 p.m. - Dinner

6 p.m. - Cleanup time followed by all lights dimmed and a quiet down reading books time

6:30 p.m. - Rocking and prayer time

7 p.m. - Bedtime

As we began to slowly help Gracin accept change as a welcomed thing, we decided that during the week we would continue to keep his life unaltered at first. However, on a predictable day for him - Saturday - we would have a new unexpected experience that would never be the same. Gracin initially welcomed this exciting new adventure. As long as we were able to discuss the outing with him beforehand all throughout the week, along with what he may feel like and how to handle the new situation, we typically had a nice excursion.

In addition to our Saturday change, during the week we started calling different family members on the phone, instead of them calling us, just because we wanted to say hi. By giving Gracin the control initially, he was able to learn that surprises can be a welcomed thing. He could then practice how he would respond if someone did this to him. He enjoyed talking and making someone's day more joyous, and, as a result, he felt good about himself.

We also wrote letters, and as old fashioned as it was, he loved it. He even began to write letters to heaven, on his own, to people we could not talk to any more. He just beamed with pride upon the completion of these small acts. He loved making someone's day and became more inclined to help another than care about his own needs. We found multiple ways to promote progress, acceptance, and love of others into our son's mind, which ever so gradually led him out of his shell more than we could have ever hoped for.

Daily we began to transform our learning hour in the mornings to not only work on academics but also social situations. We started reading *The New Social Story Book* by Carol Grey every day while we discussed each story in length. We would talk about why and how the person was feeling, what could have been done differently, and changing each story to our liking or to a situation he could better relate to. This book led us to start working more in depth on helping Gracin understand facial expressions as he learned to interpret the difference between joy, sadness, disappointment, anger, and various other emotions on someone's face. We created imaginary scenarios for him, such as receiving a gift, giving a gift, encountering someone who is crying, and how to handle the various situations. Therefore, when he gave someone a present, he was improving at interpreting the type of emotion to give back to them by seeing their reaction. Along with some guidance, this led him to start to be able to distinguish various emotions within seconds.

Even though it may seem to many individuals as silly or useless that a child needs to be taught how to express an emotion, the reality was that without instruction Gracin would have not been able to process these complex situations on his own. For only one example, crying was always extremely confusing for him. The few times that I let him see me cry, he would laugh. It was not that he thought it was funny that I was expressing my own feelings, but it was truly that he did not know how to respond to my emotions in a typical format. With reading and making our own social stories, we were able to lead our child out of a life of confusion from various emotions into a key understanding of empathy. His progress from these small one or two page scenarios was amazing as he learned how to express compassion and other emotions.

Furthermore, we started an online reading program for a very small fee, in relation to its content, called Starfall. Together we did a reading lesson a day. We found Gracin first grade math workbooks, and he also began memorizing notes to music in the form of flash cards. Our hour a day of learning was packed full of things he found fun, while he listened to various composers and jotted down the notes he believed were in the melodies.

Even though we called it nap time, rest time really became his own self-taught learning sessions as I would allow him to take in a book, a writing utensil, and a math book. We, of course, had some setbacks in the process, such as math equations being written on the wall, small chunks of that same wall being dug out with his writing utensil, and some self-exploratory behavior. After careful explanation and almost constant monitoring through the video monitor, these behaviors were controlled over the course of his 4th year as we tried our best to give Gracin what his mind craved so desperately. His brain was composed differently than most other children's, and that meant that different treatment was in order. During a time that most children would sleep for naps and also at night, Gracin spent his time writing music notes, math equations, and doing anything he could at all to fight his body's need for rest.

In his room there was only a twin mattress on the floor - for safety. During rest time, I would allow him to spin as much as he wanted, lie upside down, and just be himself for a one hour period.

In *The Way I See It* by Temple Grandin, a world renowned autistic writer, she states:

> For most of the day I was forced to keep my brain tuned into the world. However, my mother realized that my behaviors served a purpose and changing those behaviors did not happen overnight, but gradually. I was given one hour after lunch to revert back to autistic behaviors without consequence. During this hour I had to stay in my room, and sometimes I spent the entire time spinning a decorative brass plate that covered a bolt that held my bed frame together.

I related with the author that my son also needed a specified time each day to not be corrected by the behaviors that most others did not understand. Even though we were promoting growth in our child, we did not want him to feel neglected of the things that made his body feel secure, such as spinning.

I wanted to allow him to feel a sense of control over his body and actions. I did not want to change who he was! I, myself, hated feeling jittery, and because I knew what that could feel like from drinking a very sugary drink, that feeling day after day could never bring peace to anyone. Although because I believed he felt much worse than what I could from drinking too much sugar, I was left pondering how to tweak our day to allow his mind to feel secure while also giving him room to slowly accept change with each passing day.

As we have learned throughout Gracin's life, we were constantly in the process of training his mind to accept various unexpected changes. At the same time, we were also attempting to train his personality. Hence, his 3rd year was more of establishing a control over his environment. The 4th year was a training of how to interpret modification to the schedule and the accompanied feelings with those changes.

Even though we were immensely better as a family with these small changes, I felt we were nowhere near where we wanted to be. I will admit that I blamed myself. I was convinced that I could do more, read more, and prepare more. Upon feeling the walls closing in, I reluctantly forced myself time and time again to come to the realization that this child with whom I worked during every moment was never going to think the way that most children did.

Over time, I realized that I was the selfish one. I was the one who expected a child with extra needs to fit into the rigid attributes that I envisioned in my head. It may have been my job to help him learn and grow into a kind hearted adult, but it was never my job to force him to become a child with a different personality. I will admit it was an extremely delicate balance of constantly keeping ourselves in the proper mind frame without overstepping our parental boundaries.

We had to focus on the positives in our child and not let the negatives outweigh the progress we were making. Our Gracin had so many positive attributes that parents of other four year old children could not even begin to fathom. We continually worked on all of the positives we could, which for Gracin were reading, mathematics, and music. As I fine-tuned my approach to my unique child, I began to see how well he benefited.

Since we had become a family of five, counting three young boys under five who demanded a lot of attention, we, as parents, honestly were very close to exhausted at almost every point throughout our days regardless of what special needs any of our children possessed. Therefore, we explained to Gracin that each person has his or her own set of needs, and just because Gracin may, himself, feel that his needs were the most important, they were not any more special than the other members of our family. I continually explained to him that I remembered holding, walking, and rocking baby Gracin, just as I was now doing with his new sibling. As he was led to understand that everyone has their own needs, he readily accepted that he felt his brother's needs were just as important as his.

We were raising our special needs child to not feel like he was privileged by getting the attention first. Even though most times he did get the attention first, he did not need to know that was the case. Gracin was being taught to be respectful, kind, patient, cooperative, and loving. Loving and respectful were the two big words that we talked about daily. At the end of the day, he did an amazing job attempting to live out those attributes - most of the time.

Honestly, one of the hardest things for me to accept was knowing that deep inside my son's heart was a little boy who wanted, desired, and tried his hardest to listen. He loved his brothers and parents in the best ways that he could, even though he continually had a hard time expressing those same feelings. He was not a brat or a kid who loved pushing boundaries and disobeying us. His brain, frankly, just did not allow him to consistently focus on what we were asking of him. Carrying our requests out in a calm and organized manner took lots of patience on our part, which brought us to become more loving in our actions because of that fact alone.

By way of these struggles, we also helped Gracin develop compassion and service of another in multiple ways. We were always asking him to help Mommy with getting this and that or to do something for Daddy such as getting the phone or a tissue. He loved completing small requests, and it helped him feel empowered. As a result, when we would ask larger things of him,

The Life I Discovered is Ever Changing

he could listen to our request and carry it out in the exact way we requested. Sometimes we even would change our request half way through a mission, and in this way, he also slowly learned to adapt to changes in his world.

You see, I wanted my child to feel his emotions and know what to do with them, instead of letting them take over his entire world. As life moved in the direction of establishing better focus and teaching him how to love in its purest form with compassion, we all grew in the ways we needed to. Gracin is a person with feelings who desires to show them to others yet really needs extensive guidance in order to listen, follow though, and explain to others how he feels.

Looking at the totality of the 4th year of progression, I feel as though we were able to help Gracin adapt to various changes with the small, guided responsibility and tasks that we called upon him to complete. Each night, therefore, I was able to optimistically go to bed with the intention of being able to sleep eight hours continually throughout the night, and I was amazed that a good portion of the nights we actually attained this goal. Our days had bumps along the way, but as long as we could prepare Gracin before an unexpected change to his routine, life continued on with minimal perplexing issues.

Chapter 20:
Forever Imprinted

I am reluctant to admit that my husband and I have honestly talked a great deal about how we feel our son could have fared differently if he had been raised from the first moments of his life in a home with two committed parents by his side. Many questions were raised from pondering the previous thought in our late night talks about how best to help our child. If I had been free from the chaos of unpredictability in my pregnancy, would I have had all the medical problems during his gestation? As a result, would Gracin have been different, calmer, and more at peace as an infant? Would those differences have caused our child to be varied in temperament, his diagnoses, and his personality?

These questions could go on and on, and because they can and will never be fully answered on this earth, is there really even a point to their inquiries? Well, no, per se, but honestly they can become an endless spiral of emotions. To different degrees, we, as parents of a special needs individual, blame ourselves at times. We feel responsible for our child's diagnosis, and regardless if there is any point in these thoughts, they creep into our reality on a continual basis. It is a very difficult actuality of thoughts, but an article entitled "Parents Don't Cause Autism in Their Kids, and We Need to Stop Blaming Them For It" has eased my mind many times. This article appeared in *The Washington Post* on November 28, 2014, and it was written by Kristelle Hudry. What she states shows that what we were feeling was not an anomaly for our family at all:

> Since the condition was first recognized in the 1940s, parents have been and felt blamed for their children's autism. Today, most people no longer believe this, but a lingering doubt continues to niggle many parents... (In the past) Parents were blamed for their children's autism because psychoanalysts thought cold, detached parenting must be the cause of their extreme withdrawal from the social world. Some parents were seen to interact with their children in ways that were interpreted as demanding and emotionally distant, rather than supportive and warm.

There are countless articles on the internet, stories I have been told, and forceful suggestions from individuals who have proposed that maybe it was something that we were doing as parents to cause our child to act in the ways that he was. Time and time again, even though I personally knew that my child's diagnosis had nothing to do with how I was acting in raising my child, the reality, and even the unwanted guilt, remained a certainty in our lives. As time passed and I continually looked at my other children, my mind always went to question and wonder if Gracin would have fared better being raised by someone else. Even though those interactions were almost impossible not to take to heart, slowly I learned to let the comments not affect my emotions.

Facts as they remain, Gracin has truly transformed my life in a million different and vital ways because of his outright existence. I have grown not only as a parent but also as a whole person because of his impact on my life. Just a little bit of time before his conception, as I have somewhat described, I was a selfish, unrealistic, irresponsible, disrespectful, and impatient - let me say it - child. Still thankfully, with dedication, coming in contact with a few special individuals, countless nights of research, and specific tools, I was led to make all of the changes necessary for the life I now possess. A life I feel I am privileged to have. A life I feel that I am fully capable of sustaining by caring for a child with special needs.

Although our child was not an easy child in any manner, I believe that I was this child's best bet at growing to become a loving and wonderful human being in his own right. How could I be so selfish to only keep thinking of myself - my wake up call, my hardship, my...my...my! As is stated in *The Letters of Catherine of Siena*, Volume II

> In God's goodness we discover and experience charity by seeing that we have shared in this charity through all the gifts and graces we have received and are still receiving. And in knowing ourselves and sin (which we discover through that perverse law within us that has rebelled and is still rebelling against our Creator), we conceive a disgust and hatred for our selfishness. Through that hatred we discover a patience that makes us strong enough to endure pain, scorn, abuse, hunger and thirst, cold and heat, and the devil's torments and temptations; and we despise and run away from the world and all of its pleasure.

My thought process broadened as I began to open my eyes to see how I could help my son evolve and grow, instead of mistakenly and selfishly only attempting to make my life easier. I now trust that, if the saying is true, God only gives us what we can handle. If that is so, I am led to believe that God must feel I am pretty special. Raising a typical child is an endeavor in itself, but it takes a whole new level of parental commitment to care for a special needs child day in and day out. This is why I believe that God only entrusts these special children to exceptional parents.

I believe it was based on that point alone that I began to understand that in order to be that extra special parent that I believed I was being called to be, I also needed to find time to give myself a break from the constant goings of this little boy without leaving him in the hands of another person. Since I hardly ever left his presence, I truthfully needed this break more than I could describe. However, I never admitted this to anyone. I desired to be the super mom that I envisioned myself to be. I knew that I had it in me, but in reality, I knew that I had to be very careful that I did not push myself enough to break.

After much consideration and reconsideration, I came to the conclusion that I could not be the parent I wanted to be without time to myself. A half an hour a day is under four hours a week, which in proportion is significantly less of a break time than most individuals receive at a typical full time job or in combination with the drive to and from work. I feel I deserve at least that small amount of time to not be a wife, mother, or even a friend. To be just me, a human person with my own set of needs who still needed to feel as if I mattered.

I initially saved this break until the end of the afternoon nap. However, after multiple occurrences of missing out on this time and hearing Gracin running full speed down the steps, I realized that this set time had to come before all of the dishes, wash, cleaning, and dinner prep was done. So I willingly put myself first, and although I may feel guilty doing this, I still give myself one half hour a day. This refresh time is my time to do whatever I want and nothing about what needs to be done. This is a time to listen to music, write down thoughts, scream into a pillow, cry, or pray. I have done a lot of soul searching in those tiny tidbits of time, and, as a result, I am able to better help myself be in the correct mind frame to be calm and collected to keep giving my all to my child.

Of course, since life always changes, there were many times that I lost that time each day because something absolutely needed to be done that minute, or Gracin was having an off day and was screaming at the top of his lungs because we had to find a tiny fly, which could have been invisible, but nevertheless needed to be dealt with immediately. I never sacrificed my child/ren's safety for this private time, but as long as I was not extremely needed or being neglectful, I made that time a priority for my own rejuvenation.

When I lost that personal time, I discovered that instead of getting mad and feeling as if my own personhood no longer mattered, I could offer up all of my actions in caring for my child into a prayer. A prayer for my own soul's benefit or for someone whom I never had the pleasure of meeting yet had no one else to remember him or her. There were countless moments where I felt my emotions begin to get the best of me. In recognizing that I was reaching my own capacity, this was the best way that I knew to bring myself back in check.

I will admit I could have lost my mind and hurt my child in ways I would never wish to express, but this small gesture of prayer and offering or self-talk to myself was enough to clear my own anxiety. I believe that although it was never formally diagnosed, I began to have moments of situational anxiety and depression brought on by countless stressful situations. Even though I could have turned to medication for myself, I was able to bring myself out of a spiraling vortex through this constant silent prayer.

Thankfully I never resorted to physically losing myself within my own anger to abuse my child. Frankly, it was not because I was a perfectly controlled person. I am far from it, but I found self-calming resources to outlet my energy, which became the root of my prayer life.

Actually, before my words were even targeted as a prayer for help or offering, they were just a jumble of words formed out of desperation in my own head to understand how my child could possibly be arguing with me once again.

I craved, at the depth of my soul, someone to bounce ideas off of throughout the day. Since talking on the phone, going out in public, or having someone over upset my son's entire world, all that was left was myself and these little children. As much as I loved and adored my tiny people, I still craved adult conversations. I badly wanted to hear the validation that I was doing something, anything right. Even though I never felt truly alone in my heart, day in and day out in my mind, I was spinning. It was in discovering that God could also be my friend as well as my creator that everything in my world brightened up.

Within those moments, I learned to not even desire social interaction with other adults because I had found a friend who would never leave me, no matter what I cried to Him about. Those little moments, broken up throughout the day whenever I could find a few seconds, gave me the break and the restoration that my body, mind, and soul desired. I could say a simple prayer in my mind and heart such as "Please God help me not to hit my child out of anger while I explain to him for the hundredth time in the last five minutes why he cannot do... " It was because of that self-talk that I was able to stay sane.

Over time, I came to understand that this child was given to me because someone up above in the clouds - as Gracin would say at that point in his life - knows that I can handle this life. I can give this child the best care that he needs. I was entrusted and obligated to raise him to be the best little man that he could be, and that was exactly what I was going to do. How selfish could I ever have been to be thinking about the hardship that this child projected on my life by his existence? I was called to transform my desires into serving his needs in order to help him to learn, grow, and thrive in this world.

I am the first one to admit that I am NOT a saint. I do not even know if I can ever have what it takes to rise to be such an admirable being. I think of myself far too much for my liking. I screw up each and every day, multiple times per day, and I feel I rarely act in the manner that I wish to. Although, each day that I am blessed to open my eyes, I attempt to care for the child/ren with whom I have been entrusted. I ask for forgiveness from God and the little ones in my life daily when I snap and if I feel I cannot take the burdens on my shoulders. I constantly plead to God in my prayers so that I may be guided to act in the manner that I wish to model for my children.

Even though this life that I believe I have been gifted with is not an easy lifestyle, by acknowledging that, I can admit that most times basic parental needs have to be altered and sometimes outright neglected in order to optimally help an atypical child feel secure in their own needs. I can plainly admit that this is such a difficult and tricky balance that one must ultimately figure out for themselves. In knowing that fact, there are other individuals out there in the world going through a very similar situation. That fact alone should help us, as parents, never feel completely alone. Unfortunately, and at the same time thankfully, there is no manual or guide that will fit each unique child on the autism spectrum. I do believe that by elevating a person's thoughts constantly to a higher cause, I, and other parents alike, can rise above our own needs to complete what we are called to do in raising these unique children.

You see, our family was no exception from the reality of autism. The only real constant prediction that we could expect from each of our days was sporadic movement and unpredictability. However, by instilling all of the structure into our days, we were able to start somewhere. Moment to moment, we attempted to give our very best, if not more, for our child's well being. Because of this, I believe that when I look at who my son is today, standing right in front of me, all our struggles have paid off in the grand scheme of things. Our life was never easy, hardly ever calm, and without a moment that I was not correcting some type of behavior, but it has been an amazing journey that I am truly proud to call our life.

Part 6:
The Supreme Gift of Perseverance

Chapter 21:
The Magnificent Overlook

As my eyes adjusted to the brightness that surrounded us and witnessed the last few drops of rain fall upon the surrounding landscape, high upon the loft in which we were sitting, I was astounded to be overlooking the magnificent ocean from such an amazing viewpoint. With thoughts immediately bombarding my awareness, I was convinced once again that I must be dreaming; yet, I was fully awake. Could this be real? Were we finally in safety? In a true place to rest, breathe, and delight in life?

In watching the clouds dissipate around us, we could clearly see for miles into the breathtaking panoramic views that seemed to make the climb completely worthwhile. Walking closer to my son who had found a small hill to roll down, the breath left my lungs in awe. There, just ahead in the valley were more children, and they were all happily playing and interacting with my son. While observing the children spinning, dancing, and giggling alongside each other, an extraordinary peace filled me as I began to feel whole for the first time in my life.

Watching them enjoying each other's company in the sunlight, I observed them all pile on top of the man who I had stumbled upon along our journey. I could not help smiling from ear to ear.

Following after the laughter, clearing our own path deeper into the valley, we eventually came upon the security we had been searching for all along. Surveying the perfect lot of land, we excitedly began to build ourselves a home amongst the surrounding landscape.

First and foremost, we attempted to build our new valley home on a sturdy foundation, one that felt secure enough to stand for years to come. A home which housed our most precious possessions, our family of six with room to expand. Reclining back after a long day of work, I admired the grand view that I was blessed in experiencing, while in the same moment, I reflected back at all of the struggles that we had recently overcome.

Amazed at what we were capable of conquering with the help of God alone, I vowed to place my life henceforth into His hands. In my promise, I gave Him my word that although my life may at times feel out of my own control, by always remaining aware of the ocean below us and the skies above us, I would henceforth trust that with our lives in His hands we would always be led to overcome any additional storms that may be hurled our way.

Lying down in a soft bed of rose petals that had fallen to their grassy bed from the surrounding bushes, I stared up into the charming sky as the rumbles and flashes of light out in the distance were mixed among a serene pale array of colors. I fell into a dreamlike state listening to the chirping of the birds mixed with a multitude of childhood laughter. I had a hard time consciously remembering how we even came to be on this journey in the first place. Although I did not understand why I was not blessed to sit upon a calm ocean beach with some surrounding families at the water's edge, none of that any longer seemed important now that I was given the life that was in front of us. A life full of acceptance, love, stability, and peace; a life I never exactly envisioned for

The Magnificent Overlook

myself yet was the one I was led to by putting my trust in the one who mattered most of all.

♥

Life can present many difficult scenarios in our lifetimes that in the moment seem quite close to impossible to overcome. Yet, it is in those exact situations that we learn to rise above. In the pure heart of a childhood dream of the future family that I may have had, I never considered that any of my children would be anything other than adorable. Disease, physical impairments, neurological conditions, they were just something that happens to other people, not me.

Within my current world, some part of me always believed that I could do no wrong, yet as time passed I saw how childish my own actions proved to be. As it seemed, before I had my firstborn child I did not think of anyone other than myself, even though I would have argued to the end that I cared about everyone around me. Though, quite quickly all my previous thoughts changed in the months after I discovered that I was carrying a precious baby. Even though I had always believed that some aspects of my life would evolve once I had children, I never would have been able to grasp all of the ways in which I would transform at my innermost core, deep within my entire body as well as my soul.

In addition, as a woman, I felt I could predict how I would feel the first time I held my own child in my arms. I was not, however, even close to understanding the capacity of those feelings. I was not prepared for the rush of love that I initially felt for that tiny soul relying fully on my care. It was an indescribable and awe inspiring feeling to finally meet and hold a child who I had been carrying inside my body for an almost an entire year. A mother is the first to learn that they are carrying a new life, the first to hold that new life, be sleep deprived by that new life, and experience a deeper sense of love than she ever thought possible. It does not matter to the mother who that little baby will become someday or even what that child will eventually look like. What matters is that the child lying in their mother's arms is quite exceptionally perfect. The reason why a mother is so needed by their children is because of this inborn unconditional love that I believe most fathers are not privileged to feel.

A parent's attentive love and devotion is what is ultimately needed by all children regardless of age or specific condition because first and foremost a child craves to be loved. Yet in discovering and accepting that all children crave to be loved in diverse ways, our family transformed within our midst. Even though, at first, we attempted to hug our son tight, take him on unplanned fun adventures, and treat him as a typical child, we discovered that we were sending his body into sensory overload as a result.

As the weather changed and sent us running for our lives up a cold, dark, and unending mountain, we slowly found ways in which to give our child the exact kind of love that his body could accept. A love not of physical cuddles and affection, but a love based on logic and intellectually articulated truth. Yes, it was incredibly hard to change what I wanted to do for my child into what my child needed to have from me, but by accepting that each and every child is unique in their own mind, I was led to find the exact parenting strategies to calm the stormy skies around us.

Watching the skies change to only light rumbles and flashes of light as our hurricane passed and we finished climbing the mountain full of what felt like unending pain and trials, we were given the most magnificent gift. This gift was not what the world says we should desire, yet this gift was exactly what can change us all into the most glorious beings that we could ever be. A gift given to the select few individuals who are open to transforming their heart into what another needs moment by moment. A love developed by that process, I believe, is all it takes to open each of our lives to delve into the interior life of all typical and atypical individuals in order to better understand the actions at their core.

Although at times it seemed that no one else's life was harder than our own, as we were elevated to a higher level of thinking, we felt most of our earthly desires leave. In accepting that our lives may never be full of blue skies all of the time, I believe that when and if the new storm clouds roll in, we will know that not one of them will ever seem as hard now that we have surrendered our lives to a new purpose. Our eyes were eventually opened to know that our lives were not being taken from us. Instead, we learned what we could give for our child's benefit. We were led to accept that we were not failing him as parents; we were, in fact, becoming the best parents that he needed us to be within the current moment.

In the end, I feel as if we are succeeding in raising a wonderful well-rounded child who, despite his special needs, exudes joy by his presence. He may have a different way of expressing himself and a contrasting way as to what makes him feel secure and at peace, but those facts alone do not make him any less of an individual. Our son is making an amazing impact on his world to date. He excels at his school work, passionately loves his family in his own way, and inspires to become a priest to change the world one heart at a time. My husband and I could not be more proud of him, and I cannot wait to see how the rest of his life enfolds.

Chapter 22:
Other's Blunt Opinions

Some may say that I asked for this life, and in honest reality I did. In searching for my own happiness within the big wide world and by only thinking of myself at first, I became increasingly more lost with each sequential step forward. Therefore, by the own naivety of a young girl's heart, I was blindly led to believe so strongly in the wavering words of someone who told me that they loved me and wanted to marry me. I trusted fully that those words were the truth. Unreservedly, I gave that person everything, and even though I now know that by my immature thought process I set myself up for much heartache, at the time, I thought my decisions could lead to none other than a lifelong marriage filled with harmony.

However, only a few months later, sitting alone in my grandparents' back yard, on which was supposed to be my wedding day, I slowly swayed back and forth on a swing set weeping in realizing the weight of my decision that not only affected myself but also now a child. Free of all the lies and the misguidance, I slowly realized that I was now able to choose a completely new path for my life. A path chosen by transforming my devastation and tears into an unwavering strength built upon trusting in God, my supportive family, and the growing child within me. I will admit that I may have not followed the easiest course for my life by any means, yet through my budding faith, I pushed through with my dignity intact.

I had previously put my trust in another, but a being who I believed to be in the highest of the heavens freed the chains of my existence as I began to forge my straight path into the world. This path that was extremely lonely at times, but ultimately led me to the man that I believe God had always intended me to find, at the exact time I needed him most.

That man was superior to every single boy I had ever met. He was true to himself, stood for everything that I was never strong enough to vocally admit, and balanced me in all of the areas that I felt I faltered. Needless to say, he was the perfect man for me. He was the other half that would complete my life, and although it took some time for me to be able to put my full trust in his unwavering commitment, his love never faltered.

Together, we started a life based on love, one that I knew was at the basis of my being. A life whole heartily open to any new life that God chose to place within my womb to grow. As the years passed and we welcomed four children within a six year period of time, we talked continually about what we believed to be true and right within our world. Even though the match felt made in heaven, worldly obligations brought on many struggles as our son's special needs presented themselves. A child like we had been given was not easy to take into our arms, give our love to, and serve, yet that is exactly what I felt God wished of us to do.

Slowly and together we mustered the courage to rise to the challenge, and I now believe that we can most definitely be better in our responses to our subsequent struggles. We are finally on the correct path to happiness for our own family. Even though I may have been on that swing many years ago distraught at what had happened to my life, I believe that by pleading to God on that day, he lead me to the exact life he had set up for me from the moment the world began.

However, as the comments about our lifestyle began to be flooded into the interior walls of my mind, I was left swimming in a sea of emotions. As a result, I revisited that same swing set in my mind where I did nothing other than give all of whatever was happening at that current moment to God. That effort never ceased to bring comfort to my overwhelmed mind. As it states in 2 Corinthians 12:9-10, "9 'My grace is sufficient for you, for power is made perfect in weakness.' I will rather boast most gladly of my weaknesses, in order that the power of Christ may dwell with me. 10 Therefore, I am content with weaknesses, insults, hardships, persecutions, and constraints, for the sake of Christ; for when I am weak, then I am strong." By those statements alone, I became strong in love as a result of my own worldly weakness, and as Gracin's age progressed, my skin continued to get thicker. Resolving that by my weakness, God would never cease to be my strength, yet in accepting this challenge, I also had to learn to change myself in countless ways in order to help the individuals in this world view my special needs son as a gift and not a burden.

Statements bombarded us from both inside and outside of our families but the opinions within the family were inevitably the hardest to take in. Since my family believed and taught me that love, gentle guidance, and facial expressions were enough to rear a child, I quickly became the problem. As the situations escalated and a wedge was being driven between us all, the height of all the scenarios happened when my son was around three and a half. Someone very close and beloved to me decided that they had seen enough of my 'disconnected' actions to my son. Standing in my living room scolding me with their finger in my face, they expressed to me that I was the one who needed help. Needless to say, I could not find the words to argue many times as I was so caught up in my own emotionally tied feelings. As I stood there in disbelief, less than an hour after returning from church on a Sunday, I asked, through my tears, that everyone please just leave my house.

It was in that moment that I believe I once again hit a sort of bottom and my skin thickened. As I slowly rose above the person, who typically so easily fell to pieces in the moment of confrontation, I learned that I needed to acquire the words to fight for and clearly explain to others why we were parenting Gracin in the way in which we were.

The opinions had always rolled in and emotions ran high; it seemed too hard to repeatedly explain the reasons behind our actions. Our families tried their best to respect us, yet as those storms clouds hovered continually over our heads, fingers began to be pointed. I realized that our family members were struggling with their own emotions and needed someone to blame, other than a young child's neurological wiring. Sadly, I became the easiest target as an emotional response outlet. It was my fault that he was this way. I was too hard on my son. All he needed was a hug. The unavoidable responses continually radiated that he had nothing wrong with him.

Their words hurt me to my core because it broke my own heart that I could not show my child love in the way in which I desired. Yet, because of the respect I held for my own child, the person God placed in my life to raise, I would not cause him such pain because of my own selfish desires. I can fully understand that it came as a shock to most spectators that I had to be what seemed like physically detached and at the same time be more aware of my son's actions then any of my younger children combined. I felt that there was no other way around it. Gracin needed and demanded a very large portion of my attention. It was a 24/7 job that never ended, not even in the middle of the night, but one that I fully accepted with open arms.

It was exhausting, and whenever we had planned or unexpected visitors, the tensions increased because as his parents we had to be on absolute high alert. At those times he forgot all of his rules and manners in the excitement of the moment. As a result, he would get corrected increasingly more often as he had to be constantly reminded of what he was and was not to do at any moment. Viewing it all from another's perspective, I am sure that it does seem as if I overcorrected and had to 'guide', or in their words 'scold', him far too much, but our families were still only thinking of our actions in being compared to rearing a typical child.

The above scenario with one of my family member's disapproval and disgust in me as a parent did not end with that one occurrence and certainly did not end with just our family members. Everyone had their questions, comments, and advice, which were almost always the same. They just could not understand why things could not be calm, happy, and all smiles. Kids will be kids no matter what you do; no kids really listen to their parents; he will listen once he has a teacher and you are not around were some of the typical responses that bombarded our constant awareness. Though the comments just went on: if he was my child then he would listen; you just need to beat him into submission; he's just busy; time will mellow him out; he's one of those difficult children; he's just active. It was quite a spectrum of comments. My favorite was: you would not want a child that just sat there and was a blob would you?

Well now that you mention it, yes, but do not get me wrong, I would not want to trade my child for anything, but what I did want was to experience calm in my life. Children who know how to sit and play are not blobs; they are wonderful additions to a family, for they instill peace in an uncertain world. So, yes, that's all I wanted, a calm little child who played with toys and let me sit down next to them and play also. That was always the life I had envisioned having, being able to laugh, smile, cuddle, and have fun together. Unfortunately, that is not the type of child who came into our lives, and it was not an easy reality to accept but one that nevertheless needed accepting. Gracin needed parents who understood who he truly was and who could courageously stand up to help him and not ignore his problems.

So, the opinions of others continued, and aside from locking us all in the house for the rest of our lives, we eventually had to find the words to help other people also learn how to interact with our special needs child. It may not be a road easily accepted, but by showing others how to truly love, hearts begin to change over the course of a lifetime. It is tragic that in living in this world today, there are so many special needs children and adults. We need to view it as an opportunity to teach ourselves and our typical children how to have sympathy in action and feeling in order to learn how to deal with these atypical children throughout their lives.

A typical child in today's world is not going to be able to go through their life without meeting a special needs individual, and everyone should, therefore, know how to act in their presence while respecting them as the God-given soul that they are. I have had so many looks, glares, and judgments directed toward my family in public and in my home that one should never have to undergo. Even though I learned to bite my tongue and shake my head at the ignorance of most adults that crossed our paths, in hope that by my loving response they would understand how wrong they were in their accusations, the comments were never any easier to hear.

In reality, I was never proud of how strict and stern I had to be in my tone of voice towards my son, the way I had to let him cry himself to sleep when he was a toddler, or how I could not wrap my arms around him for most of his third year of life. However, I did what was best for him regardless of how easy it made my life or how it made me appear to others. I could not be the parent who everyone believed I should be. I was parenting my son in the exact way I was being called to by following his own needs.

Raising a child - special needs or not - is difficult regardless of the exact diagnosis or lack thereof, but because each situation is so uniquely different, we should all support each other in our dissimilar struggles. I would never compare my son's needs with another's. In the moment, others may think it would be easier if my child was blind, deaf, had another diagnosis that was less well known, or was diagnosis free. In reality, each person truly has no idea what that specific family is going through by raising that child. Diagnoses are not stamped on children's foreheads, and regardless of if that supposed child had a special need or not, judgments should never be made on a child or their parents for an action you may not fully understand.

Recently, there have been many opinions in the paper and the internet that speak about what causes autism. Even stating that because as little as 1% of the mothers tested in doing a certain activity, over a period of time, somehow proves that something they did caused the disorder, it can make a person's head spin. I have read that soda, antidepressants, food additives, pesticides, vaccines, parental age, prescribed pharmaceuticals for the mother during pregnancy, alcohol, and the list goes on…may inconclusively cause autism. So, for everyone out there speculating, what did that mother do to cause her son these problems, I never smoked, drank, took antidepressants, was at an adverse parental age, did drugs, or ate foods that were ill advised, and my son still has autism. I am convinced that my child inherited a genetic trait passed on in my own DNA, and until there is conclusive proof that I caused my son's diagnosis, I will raise my head high to believe that I did and am currently doing everything in my power to help my child each and every day.

Even though opinions will never cease to go away, at least it is comforting in knowing that there are numerous other individuals out there parenting through basically all of which you are. It is up to each person to find answers through doctor's offices, support groups, books, and social media. Most of what people say is only said because that person cannot fathom any way of thinking other than his or her own. If that is the case, then they are not even worth your time. Over time things do improve, and a parent starts to get a very tough skin to the comments. Even though it took me almost until my son was five to really get the feeling as if I could fight hard to get him what he truly needed, I did get to that point. This is why I believe that it is so important to slowly develop that fight and will for your child by learning to confront family members' adverse comments early on. That way, no one will ever let the infant you once held in your arms, slip through the cracks once school begins.

Chapter 23:
Becoming an Advocate

Typically as children age, they slowly detach themselves from their parents. Although the father's and mother's love never wavers or subsides, the child begins a life of independence based upon their own choices. However, for the portion of parents raising a child with special needs, life may function in a different manner. Some special needs children may, in fact, follow in the same slow detachment process of typical children. However, based upon the pliability of their needs, others may need their parents' care their entire life. As for our son's needs, we felt blessed when we were told early on that it was up to us as to the degree in which we could guide our child to function out on his own within the world.

It was indeed up to us to decide if we wanted to take the time and the commitment to guide our child through every life stage, sensitivity, and behavior, or if we wanted to ignore his quirks and just let him be him, by allowing him to act in whatever way that felt right to him at the given moment, as long as he wasn't embarrassing us. While knowing that the path we chose may have been inconvenient to the life we selfishly wished to lead, we could not find one superior reason why we should not give all of our time to help our son function to his potential.

I had much work to do with our families, acquaintances, and the world around us to become an advocate for child we were raising. I can admit that the fight did not come easy for me. As a very soft-spoken individual myself, I knew it was not going to be an easy task. I never wanted to upset any one, and in the heat of the moment, my mind always failed me. The words I wished to state barely ever escaped my mouth in the correct order. Although, it was something that needed to be done so that my son would not get bypassed. Though as a result of my own hindrances, there I was pushing my way into a brand new reality, and I felt I was being swallowed up. I knew I had to find the words to explain why I believed that our child, if given the right guidance and environment on a daily basis, could succeed in the social world. My mind willed me to develop that fight but fought with my lips as I struggled to produce the words to explain my thoughts in a manner that would not be offensive to others. With my determination and understanding, I slowly mustered the strength that I thought I initially lacked to be Gracin's best supporter without losing control of the situation.

It did require an incredible amount of time and energy, but it was not nearly as difficult as what I have found pregnancy to be. This, in turn, led me to believe that if a woman can endure pregnancy, labor, and delivery, her body and mind is already fully prepped for whatever lies ahead in the life of her child. I believe we can conquer anything for that baby who initially lies so peacefully in our arms. We just have to keep our mind and heart in the correct place while fighting for what that child deserves. It is okay to fall to pieces at home, but when fighting for the care of a child in a school setting, bring out the lawyer from the back corner of your mind to keep pushing every angle until your will is accomplished.

Becoming an Advocate

Within our own lives, by the time Gracin's fifth birthday arrived, we were only nine months away from his first day of kindergarten, and I knew we had to start preparing him for a classroom setting. Since Gracin did not desire toys for his birthday, he was basically given an office supply party to celebrate his special occasion. He asked for things like scissors, lined paper, math workbooks, word searches, and the like. He was thrilled opening all of his presents and finding these items, even more thrilled than a child getting a bike. So with our new arsenal of school supplies stocked, we began to imitate a school setting in our dining room. Each day I began to make sure he understood how to raise his hand, walk in a line, and wait his turn. He also had specified periods that I had him do his math, reading, and writing just like class periods.

In the spring, Gracin began the process of transitioning out of the early intervention. Gracin, myself, the IU physiologist, and a school psychologist from the district that our son would be attending met together in a transition meeting to discuss the ways in which we could expect life to change with the beginning of school. We discussed the services they suggested once he entered into school, and we were even given the opportunity to have those services extend into our home if need be. We discussed all of Gracin's needs and concerns, and a transitional plan was written for the school to begin with before their own individualized education plan was set up.

Leaving the meeting, I felt like we were extremely prepared for our next life stage. Within a month, we went for the first time into the school building for kindergarten registration. He met with various individuals who tested different sets of abilities, and Gracin excelled at every test. The one teacher who assessed his reading level even came up to me personally after the test to state that she was amazed by his reading level as he could read words effortlessly that most second graders would have some trouble attempting to sound out. Within the following few days, I emailed and called the head of the special education department and also the principal at the school to request testing of Gracin's abilities to ensure proper placement.

After two months of feeling as if I was battling in a one-sided fight against the school system, a psychologist from the school finally agreed to meet with us to perform a placement-type test that would assess his abilities. The morning of the test, Gracin was so excited to be back in the school building that he could not contain himself as he bounced with joy in his chair in the waiting room. After bombarding the secretary with questions, the psychologist called him into the office. Looking deeply into Gracin's eyes, I asked him to respect his words though I could see a loss of control beginning. Gracin turned midsentence and skipped excitedly behind the psychologist as the bulletproof door closed behind them both before I even had the opportunity to ask any questions. Sitting down and feeling defeated, I immediately experienced a sense of failure for not insisting that I accompany him to the test to monitor his behavior. In the back of my mind, I knew he was not prepared to control himself in an unfamiliar environment.

After only forty two minutes of a potentially two hour test, they both emerged from the long hallway, and my heart fell into pieces as I witnessed the look of overstimulation in Gracin's eyes. The psychologist seemed abnormally tense as he explained that Gracin honestly could not be controlled throughout the test. The only questions he could get him to answer were the verbal ones because he was too busy climbing on the tables and chairs while attempting to look out the window. Because the psychologist was not allowed to physically move him into a sitting position, he was not able to test his full abilities. Hearing the report, while my little boy was attempting to pull me around the room, I felt as if my heart sank into my stomach.

All the preparations we had done would be useless unless we could get Gracin to understand how to behave in a classroom setting without constant monitoring. It felt we were already in over our heads. Leaving the office that day, I was only somewhat disappointed in my son, but I was mostly disappointed in myself. I worried that by my not vocalizing his needs, Gracin's potential could not be seen. Gracin was not prepared to know how to function in a room he had never seen with a complete stranger. It was my fault for not realizing that before the testing. I lacked the strength to stand up and say what was on my mind because I did not want to feel a potential rejection. That was my fault in its entirety; although, that all changed over the next month as I found my voice for my child.

Six weeks before school was projected to start, we received an unexpected phone call from the special needs teacher at his school. She answered every question I had. I expressed to her my fears about the kind of teacher that he would need, and she assured me that he would be placed in a classroom with a teacher who could handle his needs and encourage his abilities. She was extremely nice and gave me such hope for the impending start of the school year. Hanging up the phone, I felt such peace come over my body for his first year in school. I just prayed that her superiors would not deny her requests. However, after feeling a sense of relief for a few weeks, we received the results of the intellectual test and were disappointed with the results. Given his behavior level, Gracin's reading and math abilities did not show. In fact, they were barely consistent with children of his same age. Although, it was noted that the psychologist did not feel this test showed his full intellectual abilities. Within the same week, we received another call from the special needs teacher, which added to our sadness. Almost all of her requests were denied other than being allowed to ride a special needs mini bus.

We started to feel extremely discouraged. As time passed in the wait for our final IEP meeting, I knew I had to explain that at home we had a brilliant little boy who enjoyed doing multiplication and division problems for fun, reading chapter books at a second grade level, and expressing himself by making little things, which he called art, out of scraps of paper. He thrived on school work, but I had no idea how to get the right people to see his abilities. I was unbelievably frustrated on all fronts, but I knew that this IEP meeting held the chance to advocate for our son in the ways in which I always had felt I lacked.

I had less than three weeks to prepare and prepare I did. I wrote all of my thoughts out on paper into concise responses to most questions that I imagined may be asked of me so I would not feel overwhelmed by the pressure of the situation. I took videos of Gracin doing math problems and reading his chapter books. On the day of the meeting, I brought it all along in a backpack that was crammed full of books that he had recently read, the completed math books, and the videos on my camera showing the same. Walking into the room, I felt like a college student again armed with all of my materials.

We made more strides in that IEP meeting than I could have imagined. Even though he could not be placed into a gifted program, with a little bit of persuading on our part, my husband and I made our argument why we felt skipping a grade would only benefit our son. We explained that since he was already doing more advanced math and reading, by sticking him in a classroom with children just learning the fundamentals of those subjects, we believed it would only lead him to act out behaviorally. I explained that in a more structured setting with formal desks and higher expectations, Gracin would come to know that school is serious from day one. I added that his behavior mattered more to me than his education at this point in his life, and I was willing to help as much as I could in aiding his teacher because we wanted him to start out on the best path for his school success. After providing our argument to the special needs teacher, the head of the Special Education department, the head psychologist for the district, and the assistant principal for the primary school, we all agreed that placing Gracin directly into the 1st grade program was the best course of action. My husband and I were elated with joy as we left the meeting knowing we had done right by our son. By writing down our feelings, not getting caught up in our own emotions, stating the main points in an organized and concise manner, combined with the videos and proof, we became the advocate that our son needed.

The months of worrying and fighting for what we believed was best for our child vanished as I watched my little boy excitedly wait for his bus to drive down the street. His eyes were filled with wonder while I watched him excitedly begin to enter into his new world, a new world of being without his mom for eight hours a day. Even so, questions exploded in my mind during that first fall day as his bus began to slow at our driveway.

These questions engulfed my mind as I watched him let go of both of his brothers' hands while his Daddy's hand gently held him back from running in the street when he first saw the bus turn towards us. Did we prepare him enough? Would he be able to make it through a full day of school? Would he listen? Could he control his body? Could he… Turning with only one foot on the first step of the bus he ran back to me with an excited smile in his eyes to give me one final hug and his brand new baby sister a kiss.

Smiling happily, with the sweetest moment frozen in time in my heart, I watched as he had not one ounce of fear in his body. He bravely placed his tiny foot on that big boy special needs school bus. He wore his favorite green t-shirt with green and white plaid shorts, a lanyard with his name around his neck, and his new green sneakers. Gracin greeted the bus driver with his typical slew of questions before he was interrupted to turn around for a final picture and was guided to his seat by his bus aide while he and his brothers' waved with all of their might at each other. In that moment, I was pleased with the life that I possessed. Even though it had been an amazing and difficult journey, we had completed one portion and had now begun to embark on a brand new journey starting with a memorable day of the next chapter of his life.

Less than eight hours later, my bouncy happy big boy came bounding off the bus into his daddy's arms with so much happiness it surrounded his entire persona. He could not stop talking about his day, his new teacher, all of the exciting things that happened to him, and the list just went on. I was amazed that I did not receive a phone call about his behavior on the first day, but I was ever so thankful.

Over the next few months, we were very appreciative for his teacher. She was a wonderful mix of firm and loving for him, and she started a lifelong presence of how to act in a school-type setting in his mind. She had a way with him that I do feel I know how to express in depth enough. He listened and respected her when she caught him doing something wrong. Quite honestly, she was even able to let him be himself without disrupting the other children. Slowly but firmly she guided him into what she needed while he grew immensely. As a result, he was still able to keep his happy and positive viewpoint, and we were eternally thankful for her beginning presence in his young life.

He was in school only three short months before turning six. Within those few months, we were privileged to witness exactly what we had hoped could happen with the start of his schooling. He only visited the special needs room for a few moments each day. He was excelling without much extra instruction, and his bi-weekly school therapy was in the process of ending because of how well he was responding without guidance during the school day. He had even made his first true friend. He was always so excited to begin his school day, and he was never at a loss for words in describing all of the fun things he got to do throughout his day. Honestly, I could not have wished for a better outcome, and aside from some usual imitating of others' bad behaviors, initially we did not have much trouble in those months.

Although I had struggled about which type of schooling to choose for my son, I am grateful that we initially started in the public school system. It was not an easy decision by any means given our religious viewpoints on the schooling system. In the end, because of the services that could be at his disposal in a public school setting, we had to start out with their program. With all of our heart, we wanted Gracin in a private school setting, but we had to start somewhere. I would rather see him excel and eventually be put in a private school than feel disappointed in the opposite if he could not adapt. On his sixth year birthday, marking the close of a long journey from the development from infant to school age child, I feel as if we had proved our worth as parents. We were starting to raise a child with a deep rooted moral system who is well disciplined and radiates a love for others that is beyond measure. I can stand proud and very hopeful for all our son's future endeavors and successes as he begins to leave his unique mark on the world.

Chapter 24: Confessions Straight from a Mother's Heart

We, as parents, are only given a few brief years to form a lasting impression on our young children. However, within what feels as only the snap of a finger, a parent watches their child grow into a walking and talking unique adult. The baby years flash by rapidly while they transform into the toddler years, and those change ever so quickly into the school years. It seems as if in only such a short time, those adoring eyes turn elsewhere to find what they believe the truth to be.

Parents are left behind attempting to smile at those new decisions while we are internally left longing for the baby days again. The time where just the mere presence of a mother or father could make a child grin from ear to ear. Where kisses, nourishment, and a quick nap on your shoulder were enough for a child to faithfully adore the parent's every move. Consequently, each milestone a parent experiences with that tiny child opens up the progression of a new soul leaving their mark unto the world

This alone can be a very daunting thought. In becoming a parent, we are readily given such great responsibility from the moment of each child's conception. It can seem too real, unrealistically hard, and downright scary that just one loving unifying act creates a new child. It is also a wonderful, amazing, and fascinating growth opportunity. It takes commitment, love, responsibility, devotion, and faith in order for a parent freely to give of themselves for a tiny and helpless human.

It is amazing that, as parents, we are given such an amazing opportunity to evolve ourselves and our children to grow in love, strength, passion, and responsibility by raising them in a non-wavering deeply rooted loving discipline from the moment they are born until the next generation takes over that same obligation. Forever and always that love remains, and even through the trials of upbringing, which may seem to bring a person to their knees at times, that love never subsides. These early years, although full of love, may just the same be filled with tears, trials, exhaustion, desperation, anxiety, and some bouts of circumstantial depression, which may nevertheless leave us to wonder if we are doing anything right at all.

I must admit that even though our lives did not follow the typical storybook format, over time we were led to an internal sense of happily ever after. One that may have honestly only been able to be sensed in our outward appearance once our child's small eyes were closed and his breathing finally decelerated into a resting state, it existed just the same.

Gracin, you see, was our rose among a stem full of thorns. He was not a wildflower who grew tall and carefree in a field or anywhere in which the wildflower seed touched down. He did not blow gracefully in the wind. He did not grow easily or quietly. He did not want to be sewn among countless other flowers. He was a rose, one of the most delicate of all flowers to maintain and give of their beauty.

He was abruptly placed into our lives in a bad situation with poor timing, but I believe he was placed exactly where he needed to be. I will admit wholeheartedly that we did not start out as the best parents for him. We had to grow into that role. Slowly we started to become what he needed us to be, and thankfully we were blessed with the opportunity to figure out how to help him grow into a fully blooming magnificent flower among a stem full of thorns. A rose that still may wilt when left to his own devices, though still a rose nonetheless.

One of the main things that I have learned about growing roses is that they are one difficult flower to maintain and keep in a full bloom of perfection. Between the weeds from the ground, the beetles eating the leaves, various other bugs eating the petals, the pruning of the branches, and the wind causing the delicate petals to fall to the ground, a person growing the roses can feel outright discouraged by any change in weather, temperature, or activity around their plants.

Amusingly, I once believed that you could pick out a plant from the store, bury the plant in the ground, and subsequently every single year many beautiful flowers would appear. Though as the years passed, showing a garden of basically only weeds and death, I learned that I was not very good at growing plants or flowers of any kind. It took me many years to accept and develop the proper technique to grow a beautiful garden, and, frankly, most years I still have to replant almost half of everything. Honestly, when it comes to gardening, I am lazy. I have better things to spend my time doing, and basically I just do not feel like putting in all the time to care for anything other than a few wildflower seeds.

Comparably, though, children are not something that you can just say that you do not have the time or the energy to mess with this year. You cannot throw up your hands in July and admit you're sick of raising children or disciplining them for the year. Your child cannot wait until next year for you to pay attention to and help them grow into who they are meant to be. As parents, we must persevere through the difficult times for our own child's welfare.

Consequently, I truly believe that God knew what he was doing when Gracin started growing inside me. I believe he laughed from his heavenly throne as he already knew all of my future struggles with Gracin and how I would change by the gift of his life. Nevertheless, he still chose to give me exactly him. He saw the ultimate progress in my son, the one that he will have made at his dying breath that I may never even witness. I just had to figure it out on my own, and I still need to figure it out, step by step. Oh how I wanted to know what my life had in store for me when I was a little girl, but I think it was good that I could not see it all because life is a discovery, and the best things are worth the most struggle.

Struggle I will admit we did, especially during those first five years and even though my first born son was not a cuddly little calm child who could fall asleep on my shoulder and sleep for hours, or who could sit and listen to me read him books for hours on end, or who could sit still long enough for a ten minute quiet walk in a stroller, or could sit still at the dinner table without interrupting our every sentence- to tell us multiplication equations and facts about random things that he felt was of the utmost of importance- we loved him just the same. Despite all of those things, he was, and is, an amazing child in his own right.

As is true for any child, but most especially a child with special needs, a parent must make the conscious decision to adapt and change for that child and not expect the opposite. In time, things shall be proven worthwhile, and the gift of improvement that you can witness in your own child will outweigh all of the selfish things you once thought you desired. Unfortunately, this is not an overnight awakening but a process of learning, cherishing, and accepting every individual young, old, or mentally affected, but one that, nevertheless, slowly promotes growth within each individual soul. At times, it will seem impossible and useless to even try, yet as the years unfold, parents can be led to witness vast improvements as we have.

Even though I cannot state that my child is fixed by the standards that most of the world defines as acceptable, that was never my intention or my goal. My goal was to wake up each and every morning and give my child the best version of myself that I could. Some days I will admit that I failed miserably, but at the same times that I failed him, I learned to pick myself up in the midst of my own anger, mistakes, and hopelessness and apologize to my son for my actions with the intention to always move forward and do better.

This may have been one of the hardest things to do for myself. Although by admitting that I was wrong and saying I was sorry, I taught him so much more than I ever intended to. My action became a humbling experience as I vocalized and gave my child the opportunity to understand that even an adult sometimes makes mistakes and needs to apologize when they act out of their own best interest. I want all of my children, not only Gracin, to understand that even though mommy may feel angry at their behavior, I loved and cared for them endlessly. Even though mommy may still lose control of her emotions sometimes, my love will never waver or subside.

Although it may not seem like I am cut out for this life, or that I should be caring for as many little children as I am, including a child with special needs, I believe I am in the exact place I am meant to be. I have traded in constantly obsessing with the mirror upon my wall for perfecting the interior mirror of my soul. Even though the soul may not be a physically seen object to the world around us, I believe that the mirror to my soul will do myself, as well as my family, a better endgame than any exterior mirror ever could. I have admitted that I am not perfect, but I am striving to become flawless day in and day out. Because I am not there yet, I ask forgiveness if a person has ever seen me falter in my mission.

I am certainly not writing these words to express to anyone that I have done everything right. I have acted out of anger myself and have later regretted my own emotions. I have wished that I could have taken back what I said. I have wished that the day would just end so we could start fresh again. I am even reluctant to admit that I have thought about getting in my car and never returning. Truly, I have thought some pretty horrible things, but the facts will always remain that I have never and will never act on those thoughts and do anything to jeopardize raising the children with which I have been gifted.

My husband and I have loved our eldest, as well as all of our other children, through and through it all, and we have and will always do our absolute best to help those children learn to grow and flourish. We will admit that, yes, we will each have our bad, horrible, and worst days, but we will stick with each other through all of the moments, good or bad.

We acknowledge that in order for Gracin to feel calm and controlled, we must put his anxieties and sensitivities at the forefront of our mind so that our family can function at its finest. This is why I believe I will always choose medication for my son. By caring for his mind's internal balance as well as his own mental health, we will see far greater strides in his long-term wellbeing. We will, of course, always be open to new natural treatments and medical interventions if the research is conclusive, but we will never sacrifice the progress we have made just so he can be free of the medications. I believe that although I never wanted my son on "daily pills," those prescribed medications are Gracin's best bet in balancing his brain's chemistry, which helps him to act in the ways he always intended.

No matter what choice we make for our own child, the most important choice is to choose love. Raising a child in love who truly knows how to care at their deepest capacity will leave the strongest impression on the individuals they come across in their life. I chose love over war, and although it took me some time to get to a point where I am happy to admit that this is my life, I believe that my husband and I are molding Gracin to embrace the call to love. I believe that by raising him with a big family surrounding him, with many other siblings, he will never feel alone and without true friends. That sibling bond, which can be stronger than any non-maternal friendship, is deeply rooted in their minds from the beginning of their existence.

Where there is love, trust, and hope there is always a way, and eventually with those attributes, all trials and sufferings will subside and peace will be restored to a family. Even though nothing in this life is guaranteed and life always changes, I just pray that in each family's first few years of raising their own special needs child, parents will be armed with a few good ideas or inspirations from our story. May you love with all of your being the child that God created and knit inside you from conception. Even though you may not feel it now, you are the best parent for the job of raising that child! You may have to dig deep down into your being to find the strength to make a difference in the life of that tiny child, but I believe that by that struggle, you will be led on an amazing journey of enlightenment.

I can honestly state that at times I felt I was doing a lot of things to make our lives easier instead of his better. Even if I did not have his best intentions at heart every single time, I believe my expectations of how he could transform became the basis of the best part of our lives. One full of selflessness where we promoted growth within our son that led our thought process to evolve. Where Gracin's medication became not something to keep him from hopping like a bunny constantly throughout the day but into something that could help him learn to focus for time periods when the medication was out of his system. Through knowing where we have come from and where we are now, I believe we have succeeded and will continue to in the forthcoming years.

 I may have had days where I fought with my body to get out of bed in the morning because I already knew it was not going to be calm, easy, happy, or fun. I may have had months go by where I could not call any day a good day and felt as though we would never have another happy memory in our family. I believe that it was because of those moments that I was pushed to rise above what I felt I needed to survive.

 Although life was full of nonstop battles that happened multiple times every single hour and ultimately beat me down as a caregiver, I really would never trade any of it. Even though at the peak of it all I, myself, had an increasingly difficult time being happy, even struggling to smile around my son, I came to realize that the anger I felt toward him was, in truth, really anger at myself. Deep hurt and frustrations created by my own selfishness because I could not do the things that I wanted to do anymore sometimes resulted in my feeling upset because all of my time was being spent on this tiny child. I slowly began to rise above the tears I believed were showing how much I was failing as a mother. It was during that self-expression during my private time after my children's bedtime that I found who I was created to be.

As the conclusion of this half a decade closes on my first born son's life, I am eternally grateful for who he is both on a physical level and the one at his core. On an earthly basis we have raised a child who tries so hard to be an individual who listens, cares, and loves everyone around him. Beyond his physical body, his diagnoses, his sensitivities, his anxieties, and all of the attributes that I do not have the privilege of changing, lies a soul. A soul which has been formed into a wonderfully pure entity proving everyday of a desire to become who he was created to be. A soul whom I am excited and feel blessed to witness live within the walls of my home.

My child may not be my easiest child by far, but I love and cherish him just the same, for he has taught me so much about life and love. He has given me a true passion for the first time in my life to fight for what is right for our immediate family's long-term welfare. My child is not a curse. He is not payback for all of the things done wrong in my past. He is not a burden. He is a blessing in disguise placing our family one step closer to becoming the individuals we were ultimately created to be.

Gracin, from the very beginning of his tiny presence in our lives, may have been wide-eyed, loud, vocal, and overly involved. He may have hardly ever slept, never skipped a single beat, and seemed to feed off of the action. He may have not been the least bit shy and could have cared less who you were as long as you were holding him, talking to him, or interacting with him. It may not have mattered to him if I was coming or going, as he seemed to lack an attachment to his own mother, but it was because of this child that our lives transformed into the exact ones we possess at this current moment. Facts as they are, Gracin's temperament has not really changed from day one. With our cornerstones of a strict schedule, devoutness to prayer, and perseverance, we have helped slowly mold him, and that constant, slow, and steady attempt has never been one to regret.

This child is my choice to love, and in the end, this child was my first saving grace. He may have been created from a bad decision, yet, regardless of the facts of how he has come into existence, he is a unique and wonderful addition to my family. I could never wish he were anything other than he is. I believe that everything you are given in this life is a chance to better yourself by pushing through the struggle to create a more beautiful life than you ever believed possible. Even though we may have experienced some broken wings during our five year journey, I am standing here today proud of who my son has become thus far. A mother's love knows no diagnosis, only the love for their child. Because of that fact alone it is for the love of my son and his soul that we moved beyond his autism, ADHD, and IED into perfecting our family unit on an interior level.

Appendix A: The Necessity of Sleep

Sleep may seem as if a rather redundant term within this book, yet it is such an important necessity, which many parents overlook in today's society. Nevertheless, in the culture in which we live, sleep is not viewed as important a priority as it should be. There is entirely too much stimulation, playdates, social needs, play groups, daycares, and not enough purely parent and child bonding. While it may be true that typical children can get the recommended amount of sleep without a parent's watchful eye, special needs children need their parents to be constantly aware of providing the right setting and stimulation level for the proper amount of sleep to be acquired.

Did you know that sleep is at the basis of development of the childhood mind? This is why it is imperative that a child receives the recommended amounts. Did you know that the synapses of the brain struggle to make new connections when there is not enough sleep? Did you know that children with special needs are more susceptible to sleep loss and have increased sleeping needs?

I believe the immediate family, as the norm of life on a day-to-day basis, is no longer valued as there are more and more two parent working families every year. More children are being raised

Appendix A: The Necessity of Sleep

in groups of children of the same age than ever before, and one very large negative to this way of life is that sleep suffers. Children in a daily daycare setting are woken to go to day care, limited on their sleeping in the afternoon for the entire group's benefit, and placed to bed later at night because the parents wish to see them more after work.

Even within a stay at home family's daily routine, sleep is lacking as children are awoken or put to bed later for numerous reasons such as play dates, older siblings sporting events, and social outings for the parents. Without bringing in an entirely different topic into this book, how we are deciding to raise our children in the culture in which we live is affecting our children's developing brains. They are suffering as infants, toddlers, and school age children who do not have the attention to focus on the task at hand because they are chronically tired.

It is a tragedy that many parents do not find the value of sleep in their young children's lives with the information so handily available in books such as *Healthy Sleep Habits, Happy Child* as well as numerous others. Though one thing is for sure, we need to heal our view of sleep, parenting, and the family, which in turn will heal our children at the core. I am not stating that getting the required sleep will cure all special needs diagnoses or autism, specifically, for that matter, though I believe it will dramatically help the coping mechanisms and temperament of the child. This is why I believe that sleep remains one of the most important factors for a child's mental development.

Appendix B: Toilet Training

Toilet training was not something I ever intended on including in this book, yet without it I felt I was not including everything about the first five years. With Gracin being my first child, I really had little experience with the matter. Because of that, I believe I held my expectations extremely too high. I thought that he should have been trained in the manner that I outlined for him. When that did not happen, I felt as if I was failing him and myself. In hindsight, knowing of the needs that he possessed, although unknown during his second year, I inevitably would have done so many things differently.

Unfortunately, we felt Gracin was ready because his body was able to stay dry for almost three hours throughout the day, but we never even considered that neurologically he may not have been understanding what we were asking of him. We treated Gracin like a typically developing child. Subsequently, we did many things that we felt were right, which in reality really hurt him.

We sat in close proximity while talking to him as he sat in the bathroom. We clapped and danced for joy upon his tiny drops of elimination. We used rewards as enticements for a job well done. Although, looking back on those moments in the tiny bathroom with our voices echoing off the walls, it was no wonder he never smiled back at us. Unfortunately, we had become, in those moments, his worst auditory nightmare, his worst bribing nightmare, and an emotional overload of his senses. Yes, we did toilet train him in a typical time format around age three, but it may have just been all too much and too soon for his developing mind, regardless if his body was ready.

The thought of toilet training sounded daunting for my little boy, but so did everything else in our life. We had to start somewhere, or so we thought. In noticing that he was only wetting his diaper every two to three hours, I thought I was being informed that he was getting ready for this next step. Although the task at hand still seemed impossible, given how much my child moved and how I had never done any training before, we started onto our adventure.

We set the timer for one-hour intervals, and when the timer would beep, we would have a toilet break. It took almost three months before we would have our first successful pee on the little potty and almost six more months after that, for a total of nine months, before he was going with telling us almost 100% of the time. I developed potty rules six months into our endeavor at the same time that I developed the sleep rules based on Dr. Weissbluth's book. The following are the list of rules we created:

Gracin's Potty Rules:
1. Take off your pants
2. Take off your underwear
3. Sit on the potty
4. Pee and/or poop
5. Wipe
6. Put on your underwear
7. Put on your pants
8. Flush the potty

Appendix B: Toilet Training

9. Wash and dry your hands

10. Good Job - Reward: You get to play with your potty toy!

The written rules posted in our bathroom worked really well, and over time we would discover that seeing the written words made him cooperate with us so much more easily than what we previously expected. He enjoyed having the words read to him repeatedly upon entering the bathroom. Although, at the time it felt silly to write out rules for such a young child to comprehend. Since we discovered his language ability taking off at such a young age, we felt this worked best for him. I think that the only reason he really picked up on in it in a year and one month was because of the repetition and the rules that I established without even really knowing what I was doing.

One month after he turned three he was fully trained with no accidents. We felt so empowered with what we had achieved with our child, and I believe it was because of the consistent routine that we stuck to in order to accomplish the task at hand. One thing I could never understand before he was fully trained was why he had such fear in his eyes when he was attempting to eliminate on the potty. I also could not understand the way that he looked at me when I clapped with joy and danced to show how proud I was of him. What only perplexed me all the more was that he had no smile, no emotion, nothing but fear in his eyes, which is why I would never recommend beginning training with any child who may seem skeptical to the act of training. In time, mostly all children become toilet trained, and being patient with your child is more important than who among your friends trained their child first. Think of your child's emotions first and foremost before anything else. They will thank you in time.

Appendix C: Family Explanation Letter

-As of Friday March 23rd, 2012 our son has been officially diagnosed with ADHD, High Functioning Autism, and Intermittent Explosive Disorder.

-Gracin has been seen by three professional doctors, including a psychiatrist who has officially diagnosed him.

-Although he is young, the doctor administering his new medication feels that he will have a better start on life if he is treated now. His medication can then be balanced correctly before he starts school in a few years.

-We were told that we are doing the best thing for him by keeping him on a consistent routine with predictability and certainty that he can count on in his daily life. The doctor was very happy to hear that I am staying home with him and that I do not leave the home for work on a daily basis. She told us that what he needs right now is one person who provides all of his care and needs on a consistent basis, so babysitting will be limited for a while.

- We are going to do the best thing we can for him. By giving him such a predictable schedule, we are easing his mind. As of now, he distinguishes his days by our tight schedule where he can always predict what is coming next. He also understands that on Saturdays we do something fun as a family when Daddy has the whole day off. Sundays we visit family. Usually if this daily routine has a disruption, he does not handle the change easily, and it can lead to a meltdown.

The diagnoses were given because:

- ADHD: He has such a hard time focusing that he cannot sit still for any period of time. He cannot play with a toy for more than thirty seconds without constant prompting, and he is easily distracted.
- High Functioning Autism: He has a very difficult time understanding social cues and understanding personal space of others. He also is highly intelligent and above his age level in learning his letters and reading words as well as numbers, and he is already multiplying numbers.
- Intermittent Explosive Disorder: He has a hard time handling thoughts that pop into his mind without acting on these thoughts, even if they may potentially harm him in the process. Also he shows aggressive behavior, which he does not understand as being harmful, towards adult family members as well as other adults who try to give him simple commands or tasks.

The medications that he is currently on are as follows:

- _____ for his anxiety which helps him to process his aggressive thoughts caused by the intermittent explosive disorder, instead of acting on those thoughts in an abrupt and hurtful manner.
- _____ is to control symptoms of attention deficit hyperactivity disorder which are for difficulty focusing and acting on impulse as

Appendix C: Family Explanation Letter

well as remaining still or quiet when compared to other children who are the same age.

- _____ which is a natural sleep aid to help him fall asleep quicker and stay asleep throughout the night.

Reasons we chose to put him on the medications now:

For ADHD:

- He will have a better ability functioning in his daily life if he has the attention to sit still and be able to focus on his learning, schoolwork, and teachers.

For High Functioning Autism:

- Since there are no medications to treat autism, therapy sessions will be held inside our home on a weekly basis for as long as they are needed and will then continue at school if they are deemed necessary. The earlier treatment is started, the better chance he will have reacting well in social situations that will arise soon in school and in life.
- Because he is so young we can help him relearn behaviors that he has learned to act on that would be harder to change as he progresses in age.

For Intermittent Explosive Disorder:

-Our son proves to be a very sweet little boy when his feelings and impulsive actions are not taking him over. We want to teach him that he does not have to act on these impulsive thoughts that pop into his mind.

- This disorder can get a lot worse as he gets older, if it is left untreated.
- It is commonly known as "rage" in adults, which shows signs such as acting on a quick impulse, that he does not even remember because his brain was moving so fast or that he did not intend to even do such an action in the first place.
- We have already seen this behavior when he kicked Grandma in the chest repeatedly when she was watching a movie with him, and we had to physically restrain him.
- As of right now his aggressions are controllable because he is still so little. We can pick him up and restrain him to keep him safe, but as he gets older, this will be harder to do because he will be able to fight back more.

Our Plea

We would graciously appreciate if you could go along with the treatments that we have outlined for Gracin and understand that, as his parents, we are doing the best thing we can for him. We are giving him all the love and respect that we can, in the best way that his body can best process, along with getting him the help he needs. We are providing him with the rules, structure, and discipline that will help him grow into the well-rounded individual that we know he can be. We understand that everyone has concerns and would like to help us with what we need, but, at the same time, please understand that we see him on a daily basis, and thus far we have been able to provide him with all of his needs. We will ask for help if and when we feel overwhelmed, if it is in HIS best interest.

We also know that everyone is concerned with his behavior towards other children and mainly his baby brother. I want to reassure everyone that we have not seen any behavior that leads us

Appendix C: Family Explanation Letter

to believe that with a constant eye on him, he will be a threat to any child. He has only ever shown normal jealously issues in the past and loves his brother more than we could have ever hoped for.

Lastly, we have heard remarks that many of you wish you could help us by taking him for a few hours or for the day, and while we appreciate the gesture, please understand that our main intention is to give our son a consistent person with him at all times so that he cannot bend the rules and get away with actions that another person, other than his mother, may let slide. NO ONE SHOULD EVER LET GRACIN'S BEHAVIORS SLIDE BECAUSE HE WILL THEN FEEL THAT IT IS OKAY TO ACT ON THEM! Please be assured that we do get a break when he goes to bed at night and during his nap/rest time in the afternoon. We realize that the best way for him to function well in his life is for us to make these sacrifices now and help him the best way that we can with professional support.

Thank you for your cooperation!

Please feel free to alter this letter for your own family's specific situation.

Appendix D:
1st Week of Medication

March 26th- Was given his natural sleep aid at bedtime and fell asleep within fifteen minutes of taking the medicine (compared to hours, as before). He woke up three times (compared to a norm of every hour) during the middle of the night screaming for us, but he was able to fall back asleep within seconds of us going in to get him. He woke up at 7:00 a.m. the next morning. He had the first dream that he ever remembered.

March 27th- Was given his two medications in the morning following breakfast. We had trouble getting him to swallow the medicine. After an initial panic where we thought he chewed the pills, we found them under his tongue. Tried whipped cream, ice cream, and honey to help him swallow the pills. We noticed no change in his behavior in the morning. He did not take a nap and still proceeded to kick the wall for the entire nap time and/or drummed his stomach for the whole two hours, although his mouth was quiet. Fell asleep after taking the natural sleep aid and slept until almost eight a.m. for the first time EVER.

March 28th- Took both pills after a big breakfast at 9:00 a.m. Behavior in the morning was amazing. He pulled all of my mixing bowls out of the kitchen cabinet, and before I could correct what I thought was a destructive behavior, he proceeded to his ball pit where he filled up his bowls and asked his baby brother if he wanted some food. I watched in awe, for this was the first time that my children were not only playing together, but they were also interacting and sharing. As I sat on my kitchen floor for the next two hours, I witnessed the greatest miracle that I had ever seen in person. My son was actually playing with toys. He was not only playing with them, he was also creating a game out of his own imagination and focusing on these five bowls and twenty-some balls. He transferred those balls throughout those bowls as he pretended to make a variety of different foods for his baby brother. Even through his appetite was more limited during the morning and through lunchtime, he was very kind and extra polite as he sat in his booster seat while we ate together without much correcting to sit still. He rested in his bed with no loud noises for two hours. He was in a great calm mood all afternoon with no jittery movements. He fell asleep at 6:30 after the natural sleep aid at 6:00 p.m. This was the first night where he slept through the entire night with NO screaming out in the night.

March 29th- Woke up at 7:00 a.m. and took both pills after breakfast at 8:00 a.m. Behavior was great again in the morning; he played by himself with toys. His attention was held on those toys for at least ten minutes each. I feel like I have a new child! Ate great at lunch. Said he was tired, but he could not sleep at nap. He was quiet again for two full hours in his bed. Great again after nap, but he did have a big tantrum when I said "No" to him around 4:30. He was good through dinner, but around 5:00, we saw his drumming, stuttering, and running slowing reappearing and increasing as bedtime approached. Sleep aid at 5:45. He was asleep by 6:00 p.m. Woke up three times screaming again but was easily put back to sleep within a few moments of entering his room.

Appendix D: 1st Week of Medication

March 30th- Woke up at 7:30 a.m. Took pills at 8:00, and by 9:00 a.m. he was acting calmer and wanted me to read him books. My grandparents came over for a planned visit and stayed for an hour. He did not jump on them, and he listened calmly when they asked something of him. I also had an important phone call with the doctor to update her on his first few days on the medicine. He played quietly on the floor by me for the entire phone call. He ate a good lunch and then FELL ALSEEP for two and a half hours. Acted very calm through dinner. Started drumming himself around 5:00 p.m. He fell asleep at 6:30 p.m., twenty minutes after the natural sleep aid.

March 31st- Woke up at 8:30 a.m. and took his pills after breakfast. About an hour later, we started to see the effects of the pill start, but he kept drumming his body all day. He was calmer than before he started medicine but not as much as the previous days had been. Ate barely anything all day. Took a two hour rest, but never fell asleep. Bed after the natural sleep aid at 6:30 p.m.

April 1st- Up at 7:30 a.m. and ate a quick breakfast followed by his medicine. In the car by 9:00 a.m. with a huge tantrum because I forgot to warn him last night that we had the doctor's appointment. Talked and drummed himself incessantly for the duration of the car ride. After meeting with the doctor, she gave him his first increase in dosage, but she was very impressed with his new found ability to play and progress.

Appendix E: Sensory Integration Therapy

Sensory Integration Therapy, which is a form of occupational therapy, targets the senses of an individual in specific ways in order to desensitize the accompanying heightened and overwhelming feelings that children with autism can experience. To an autistic individual, this can be the key to success or failure in living out in the world, yet it is still not a well-known practice. Few occupational therapists even offer the service because it is not looked at as a necessity. Although as a parent raising a child with sensory needs, I cannot fathom why anyone would pass up the opportunity to make their own child's life more easily tolerated.

Looking back on my own son's life, if I had known that I could help restructure his sympathetic nervous system by brushing his body multiple times per day in a certain way with a specially designed therapeutic brush, I would have done it. If I had known that I could have taught him to welcome my hugs by providing deep even pressure all over his body multiple times per day, I would have done it. If I had known about sensory specific games, relaxation therapy, and all the numerous learning experiences that come from sensory integration therapy to alleviate my son's fears and feelings that seemed obscure, misunderstood, and strange, I would have taken any such measure to alleviate his painful sensations from the earliest moments that they were recognized.

Sadly it took until after the start of my son's 6th year to be enlightened to these therapies, but if only I had known, I would have included it in our weekly appointments. May the value of this specialized sensory integration therapy, a subset of occupational treatment, become better known as places such as Schreiber Pediatric in Lancaster County, Pennsylvania continue to reach out to individuals all over the world. With your child's best interest in mind, you can conquer their largest needs, provide them with immense amounts of care, and deliver them an easier life, but it is dependent upon the choices that you decide are of the utmost importance. May you be up to the challenge!

References

Attwood, T. (2008). *The complete guide to Asperger's syndrome*. London: Jessica Kingsley.

Ball, J. (2008). *Early Intervention & Autism: Real-Life Questions, Real-Life Answers*. Arlington, Tex: Future Horizons.

Deweerdt, Sarah. (2014, November 24). Genetics first: A fresh take on autism's diversity/ spectrum – autism. Research News. Spectrum. Retrieved from https://spectrumnews.org/ features/ genetics-first-a-fresh-take-on-autisms-diversity/

Diagnostic and statistical manual of mental disorders: DSM-5. (5th ed.). (2013). Washington, D.C.: American Psychiatric Association.

Grandin, T. (2011). *The way I see it, Revised and Expanded: A Personal Look at Autism & Asperger's*. Arlington, TX: Future Horizons.

Gray, C. (2010). *The New Social Story Book, Revised and Expanded 10th Anniversary Edition*. Arlington, TX: Future Horizons.

Hudry, K. (21 November 28). Parents don't cause autism in their kids, and we need to stop blaming them for it. Retrieved from https://www.washingtonpost.com/posteverythingwp/2014/11/28/parents-dont-cause-autism-in-their-kids-and-we-need-to-stop-blaming-them/

Little Catholic Bubble. (2011, October 17). Why I never should have had eight children. Retrieved from http://littlecatholicbubble.blogspot.com/2011/10/why-i-never-should-have-had-eight.html

Laura, Curran, Craig Newschaffer, Li-Ching Lee, Stephan Crawford, Michael Johnston, and Andrew Zimmerman. (1 December, 2007). Behaviors associated with fever in children with autism spectrum disorders. *Pediatrics*.

Montessori, Maria. It's more than just fun! Child development & play are related. Play Is The Work of the Child" Child Development Institute. Retrieved from http://childdevelopmentinfo.com/child-development/play-work-of-children

Noffke, S. (Trans.). (2001). *The letters of Catherine of Siena* (Vol. 2). Temple, Arizona: ACMRS Publications.

Noffke, S. (Trans.). (1980). *Catherine of Siena: The dialogue*. Mahwah, New Jersey: Paulist Press.

Notbohm, E., & Zysk, V. (2012). *Ten Things Every Child with Autism Wishes You Knew: Updated and Expanded Edition*. Arlington, TX: Future Horizons

Popcak, G., & Popcak, L. (2010). *Parenting with Grace: Catholic Parent's Guide to Raising almost Perfect Kids*. Huntington, Ind.: Our Sunday Visitor.

Starfall: Learn to Read with Phonics. (2002-2015). Retrieved from http://www.starfall.com

Timing of the Diagnosis of Attention-Deficit/Hyperactivity Disorder and Autism Spectrum Disorder. (2015). *Pediatrics*, 136(4).

Toddler Sleep Issues? My Tot Clock is the first all-in-one Toddler Sleep Clock, Toddler Activity Management Tool. (2008). Retrieved from http://www.mytotclock.com

Weissbluth, M. (2003). *Healthy Sleep Habits, Happy Child: A step-by-step program for a good night's sleep* (3rd ed.). New York: Ballantine Books.

Wojtyla, K. (1993). *Love and Responsibility* (Revised Edition ed.). San Francisco, California: Ignatius Press.

About the Author

Janele Hoerner lives with her husband and their soon to be five children in Lancaster County, Pennsylvania. She loves every moment she has as a stay at home mom where she has found her greatest fulfillment. Janele awakens each and every day as she works to guide all of her children to learn and grow in love for another while they discover the world around them. She especially attempts to guide her first born son on his journey of living day in and day out with the multiple diagnosis' of High Functioning Autism, ADHD, and Intermittent Explosive Disorder. She teaches him daily with her words, guidance, and love that his diagnosis are important for others to understand why he is different, but his soul in which she believes is buried beneath the diagnosis itself will only define him.

Three years ago, while sitting in church, she received an inkling that she was additionally being called to help other families navigate through the waves of discovering their own child's special needs diagnosis. In being a very private person herself, she at first felt that she was not up to the challenge. Now that book has come to fruition in the form of *Loving the Soul Beneath the Autism*. Her only hope is that she can help just one family who is struggling in the same battle that she and her husband did with their first-born son. Her wish is that the soul of each and every human person, created equally by God, may be loved and rightfully respected for his or her own unique impact on this earth.

You may contact her at:
lovingthesoulbeneaththeautism@hotmail.com
facebook.com/lovingthesoulbeneaththeautism
lovingthesoulbeneaththeautism.com

Made in the USA
Middletown, DE
31 March 2016